AD/HD GENERATION

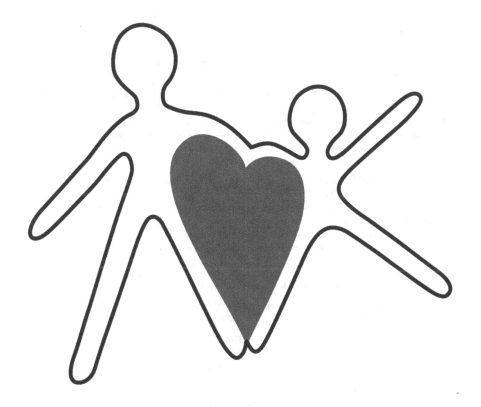

Holistic Ways to Support Children

Cecilia L. Lopez Zúñiga Ph.D.

Order this book online at www.trafford.com
or email orders@trafford.com

Most Trafford titles are also available at major online book retailers.

Cover Design/Artwork by: C. L. Lopez Zúñiga

Photography (for author photo) by: R. O. Bumpass

Note for Librarians: A cataloguing record for this book is available from Library and Archives Canada at www.collectionscanada.ca/amicus/index-e.html

Printed in Victoria, BC, Canada.

ISBN: 978-1-4251-8114-7 (sc)
ISBN: 978-1-4251-8115-4 (e-book)

Our mission is to efficiently provide the world's finest, most comprehensive book publishing service, enabling every author to experience success. To find out how to publish your book, your way, and have it available worldwide, visit us online at www.trafford.com

Trafford rev. 9/2/2009

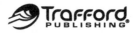

www.trafford.com

North America & international
toll-free: 1 888 232 4444 (USA & Canada)
phone: 250 383 6864 ♦ fax: 812 355 4082

Dedication

This book is lovingly dedicated to my precious Mother,
Dora Alicia Lopez Zúñiga, with the deepest of gratitude.
It is because of her belief in me
and trust in Grace that this book exists.
May it serve as a guide to those seeking to be for their children
what my mother is to me:
a lifeline of support, faith and love.

■   ■   ■

Acknowledgements

There are many people who deserve thanks and gratitude for their role in creating this book.

So much love and gratitude go to Lorri C.J. Rivers, for creating such an aesthetically and energetically beautiful space for me to write, for supporting and motivating me during times of frustration, and for holding me steady during the final phases of this book's completion. To you, I offer my deepest thanks, love, and the smile in my heart.

My sincere thanks and gratitude go out to the family, friends, and professionals who gave their time to read and edit early versions of this book. Extra special thanks go to Beth Powell, LCSW, and Dr. Arturo Volpe, as well as to friends Lisa Calgaro, Lynne Schaffer, Cindy Judkins, and Joyce Jean for their persistent and loving support. Special thanks also go to Bill Morgan and Trisha McWaters for their role in launching the initial formulation of this book.

Table of Contents

Appendices

INTRODUCTION

ATTENTION-DEFICIT/HYPERACTIVITY DISORDER, OR what we now call "AD/HD," has been a hot topic of conversation among parents, educators and all types of health professionals for many years now. It exploded into the number one position for children's diagnoses in the 1990s. Suddenly, everyone thought their child had it, and very rapidly, millions of children were diagnosed with it. AD/HD is just one of many diagnoses that are given to children as young as two years of age these days by psychologists, psychiatrists and physicians. Following diagnosis, the vast majority of children are placed on some type of prescription medication to "control the symptoms." And that is why I chose to write this book.

As a Licensed Specialist in School Psychology in Texas, I worked with hundreds of these kids in the public schools. I assessed their language, intelligence, achievement, history, general health, and social-emotional functioning to help with decisions about their needs at school. I was also their "Special Education Counselor" to help them heal emotional wounds, find successful coping strategies when stressed or to learn new social behaviors. So, I got to know these kids on a very personal level and I got to see the world through their eyes. I also worked with many of their parents to help them find ways of supporting their kids while getting done what needed doing in more harmonious ways. So I got to know their families, as well.

From this position, I had access to the kids' school, home, personal and social lives. I got to see the kinds of things they were good at and the kinds of things they struggled with. I got to know what things helped them succeed, and what things kept them from being and doing their best. My goal has always been to find the things that help kids be and do their best, and then try to fill their lives with them. I believe that we are all capable, lovable and valuable, and I believe that kids will show us just *how* capable, lovable and valuable they are when given the room to do so.

I chose to write this book about children's symptoms because I am disturbed by how quickly the number of kids with psychiatric diagnoses skyrocketed in the last 15 years, by how young the children are when they are placed on high-powered prescription drugs, and because I have serious concerns about how we, as a society, have chosen to view and deal with children's behavioral symptoms. In this book, I focus on AD/HD since it is one of the diagnoses that is given most often to youngsters, but there are others that can be viewed in the same way.

My concern for children today, and especially with the creation of what I call "the AD/HD Generation," is that rather than taking the time to nurture their wholeness, we are, as a society, letting go of our long-term responsibility to them. We are forcing children into rigid categories of "diagnosis," abandoning nurturing for pharmaceutical drugs, and expecting them to continue to function. With AD/HD, we have created an entire generation of children whose primary wellness tool is prescription drugs. Twenty years ago, it was almost unheard of to give children prescriptions like we do today. Why has this happened? We could speculate a thousand different reasons. The question in my mind is no longer why it happened, but how do we shift it to something healthier for children in the long term?

As it stands, professionals and parents alike are divided in their views of what AD/HD is, what causes it and how we should treat it. There is so much information out there about this diagnosis; it can be very confusing for parents when trying to make decisions for their children. I'm hoping that this book will help clarify some of that information for you.

I am also hoping that this book will create an opening of conscience in your mind, your heart, and in the neat packaging we've created around AD/HD. There's so much room for questioning and discovery in this area of our children's lives. I believe we should keep talking about it until we, as a society, can feel unified and good about how we deal with it. There's no question that the symptoms we call "AD/HD" are real. They're life changing and affect children, adolescents, adults, families, and classrooms alike. They are not to be ignored; just revisited.

How is this book different?

You may be thinking: "How can this book tell me anything that I haven't already heard about AD/HD?"

This is *not* just another book about AD/HD. This one is different. It is a resource guide for parents who aren't sure about using drugs to shift their child's behavior. It will tell you enough to make some immediate changes in your child's life, and to make an informed decision about how to deal with their wellbeing and behavior in the long run.

The truth is that there is still a lot we *don't* know about AD/HD. Most of what we've learned over the past 100 years has led us to more questions. Researchers, doctors, and people who work with children don't agree on what AD/HD is, what causes it, or how to treat it.

These are the questions that I cover more thoroughly in the *AD/HD Generation Companion Book* to this guide. (For an extensive discussion of the research on the pros, cons and controversies surrounding the AD/HD diagnosis and using drugs as treatment, refer to the *AD/HD Generation Companion Book*). Yet, despite all the information out there, you may still have a lot of questions about how to best deal with your child's development. In Part I of this book, I review the findings that led me to question our current approach to children's symptoms, and I propose a shift in the way we view children's functioning. In Part II, I discuss what you can do to maximize your child's long-term wellbeing while addressing their development without using questionable drug treatments.

It's clear to me that the health care model we've been using to support children's development– known as the "medical model" – isn't working very well. It doesn't seem to be creating healthier children, even though we've used it for years to handle their "AD/HD" and other symptoms. The medical model assumes that if people's symptoms "look" the same, they must mean the same thing and can be treated in the same way. It also assumes that most health problems can be fixed with drugs or surgery.

I believe that our histories, bodies, and lives are too individual and diverse to use this type of "blanket treatment approach" to address symptoms in a healthy way. And I also believe that kids' developing bodies are too vulnerable to be pumped with strong prescription medications that alter their blood, brains, neurotransmitters, and hormones when other helpful choices are available, especially when the drugs have so many risks attached to them and questionable long-term benefits.

Instead, I say it's time to view children's health and ability to function from a more complete model of health care that considers their uniqueness and aims for healthy, long-term growth rather than quick, short-term (temporary) changes. This is like the difference between putting a bandage over a festering wound, and treating the wound for infection. If you simply put a new bandage on every day, new skin may grow over the wound and it might look healed from the outside, but in the long-term, the wound will start to show new signs of disease. However, if you treat the wound for the infection, it might not look very pretty on the outside at first, but it will be healing from the inside out, and in time, that area will recover.

We can view kids' behaviors as symptoms or indicators of something out of balance in their body or being (a "wound"). We can either give them a pill to make it appear better on the outside (put a bandage over it) or we can find ways to bring them back into balance (treat the infection). In my view, our goal with children is to heal them on the inside so that they can grow and glow on the outside with full, long-term health and success.

The alternate approach I suggest in this book is known as the "holistic model." The holistic model says that health is the result of a lot of different things in combination with the uniqueness of your child and his or her body. Within the holistic model, your child's body, thoughts, emotions, spirit, lifestyle, experiences, and environment are all seen as important parts of their overall wellbeing and ability to function. Symptoms are seen as a sign that there's an imbalance in one or more of these areas. Each area is looked at as a possible place to focus treatment.

Treatments used by holistic doctors can include many things, like changes in some part of their "environment" at home or school, dietary shifts, lifestyle changes, emotional work, bodywork, or even natural medicines. If prescription drugs are used, it is generally as a last resort or when the body seems to be in crisis, because prescription drugs tend to work faster than natural medicine (which is what you want when in a crisis).

As you read this book, it's my hope that you will find the information you need to make clear decisions about what's best for your child's long-term health and wellbeing. With so much information out there about "AD/HD," deciding what to do can be frustrating, scary, and hard for parents. This book is meant as a resource guide for you, to help you decide how to best support your child in being their best every day and in years to come.

In this book you will find:

- Current and comprehensive information about the pros, cons, and controversies of the AD/HD diagnosis

- Reliable information to help you make your own decisions about holistic choices

- Exercises, examples, tables, lists, and charts to help you make decisions and changes more quickly and easily

- Resources that you can check out for more information

What I ask you to remember while reading this book is that I am sharing my personal views, opinions, and experiences with you, as well as those of many other professionals and researchers who work with children. You may not agree with all that you read in this book, and that's OK. I don't expect you to, and I don't want you to take what I, or anyone else, say as the absolute truth. The ideas I share in this book can be accepted as truth only to the degree that they are certainly true by the beliefs of some people. No one, and certainly not I, can claim to have all the answers to the puzzle of our children's health and wellbeing. Each person must form their own opinion of what is best for their child based on their own personal belief system, values, experiences, ethics, and whatever information they have access to at the time. I believe that the more information you have, the better able you will be to make up your own mind about what approach will work best for supporting your child.

This book is simply one more piece of the very large AD/HD puzzle. It is a piece, though, that can't be ignored. For, however small a puzzle piece may seem or however much we may want to discredit or ignore it, each piece is needed to complete the whole picture. The information I share in this book is meant to support you in your search for the complete picture of this puzzle for your child. Your willingness is all that's needed to make the journey with me. Happy Trails!

PART ONE

TAKING A SECOND LOOK AT AD/HD

1

THE WHATS, WHYS AND HOWS OF AD/HD

History, Causes, Controversies, and Treatment Issues

Why Revisit AD/HD

MOST PARENTS HAVE heard of Attention-Deficit/Hyperactivity Disorder, or "AD/HD." Most of us have heard these words *so* many times that we cringe when we hear them now. It seems that there are hundreds of books on the topic, and there are now over 7 million children with the diagnosis.

Let's say that your child is diagnosed with AD/HD. You're probably coping with challenging behaviors every day. Your child may be having repeated problems at school. I bet you want to *do* something, but you're not sure what. Everyone you talk to has their own ideas about what's best, and they don't always agree. You want the problems to stop. It can be draining on your family. You may be a parent who is called to the school over and over again because your child has done something that's not allowed there. You may have a child who gets suspended and sent home for several days. Then, you must figure out how to care for them and get to work at the same time. It may put your job at risk. This can be very stressful. You may feel frustrated, embarrassed, guilty, ashamed, scared, mad, sad or confused about why this is happening.

The AD/HD diagnosis gives parents a reason for their child's behavior and the struggles it can create within a family. Parents can stop wondering what they're doing wrong and rest in the knowledge that their child "has" something that can be treated. Parents can also sigh a sigh of relief at having a starting point for change. Diagnosing a child as having AD/HD generally leads to understanding and support from others, treatment choices, and most importantly, some genuine solutions. For some parents, this means that their search for an answer can end. They can start to deal with their feelings around it and begin doing things to change the situation.

As a school psychologist, I've seen the symptoms we call "AD/HD." I've worked with hundreds of kids who were diagnosed with it. I've talked to their parents and teachers. I've seen how the symptoms can impact a child's learning and relationships. At first, the AD/HD diagnosis gave me a place to start my search for understanding and help. The AD/HD label gave struggling children access to special services in the schools. Experts who cared about children felt it was helpful and necessary, and so did I. I still believe that the AD/HD diagnosis may be helpful and necessary for a small subgroup of these youngsters, but for most of the children we label as "AD/HD," I believe we are off track.

Over the years, something began to change in the schools. The number of children diagnosed with AD/HD exploded in the 90s, and we started to look at behavior differently. Lines of students formed in the hallway outside the nurse's office during lunchtime, waiting to get their "AD/HD meds." If a student diagnosed with AD/HD was darn near anything but perfect, adults asked, "Did you take your medicine today?" More and more, teachers and other adults began saying to me, "This child is very difficult. I think (s)he has AD/HD." This became the norm, instead of taking a thoughtful look at all the things that can be a part of a child's ability to succeed academically and socially.

Of course, part of diagnosing a child with AD/HD means that certain things must be "ruled out" as not causing the behavior. "Screenings" are done to check for this. The areas screened include:

1. health issues (vision or hearing weaknesses)
2. language difficulties or differences
3. a lack of schooling or interruptions in learning opportunities
4. severe emotional issues from family or other stressors

5.   low intelligence
6.   learning difficulties

The problem is that much of the time, the screenings are too broad and non-specific to pick up all the things that could affect a child's behavior in ways that might create AD/HD-like symptoms. As an example, consider the student who has a severe vision problem – not the kind that leads to blindness, but the kind that has to do with how the eyes work together – like problems with visual tracking or eye teaming (See "Links Between Sensory Input and AD/HD Symptoms" in Chapter 9). Students can pass the standard eye chart used for vision screenings and still have a serious vision weakness that isn't identified. This weakness can lead to unhealthy coping behaviors that we label as "AD/HD" in a child. As another example, consider the child who has an allergy or sensitivity to a food such as corn that hasn't been identified. That child will behave in ways that can look like what we call "AD/HD" every time (s)he eats that food, yet there is nothing specific in the testing process that screens for nutritional issues. I believe that continuing to downplay or ignore "loop holes" such as these in the assessment process for diagnosing youngsters with AD/HD is doing them a disservice.

I've also found that by the time testing begins, many people's minds are already made up about a child. The behavior checklists parents and teachers fill out describing a child are easily "stretched" to fit their views, and presto! Just about any child can look "AD/HD." It all depends on how adults rate them. For the person doing the evaluation, there are few checks for truthfulness in how kids are rated, except by comparing the ratings of the different adults, like parents and teachers, and having other checks in place, like watching the child yourself.

Getting ratings from different people who see a child in different settings is supposed to help prevent "automatic" diagnosis, but...people talk. They talk about how they see a child and what they think he or she needs. They talk about what can be done for the child and how to get it done. They talk from experience or concern or exhaustion. They talk from a wish to help. Whatever their reasons, they often talk to get agreement.

If you want to, you can make almost any child fit the criteria for a diagnosis of AD/HD. It's not hard to do. The behaviors are traits that we *all* show to some degree. Where someone draws the line between average and abnormal behavior is a very personal decision. For example, saying that a behavior happens "All the time" might mean four times an hour to one person and eight times an hour to another, yet both might see this as quite normal. Someone else might believe that three times an hour constitutes "All The Time" and is abnormal. So, how a child's behavior is rated on a scale is highly dependent on the beliefs and views of the rater.

For all the research that's been done, we still don't have a test that finds AD/HD. What *has* been shown is that the "observe and report" methods we use to diagnose AD/HD today aren't reliable enough to tell the difference between abnormal and average behavior. They also don't give us any idea about what is causing the symptoms (or behaviors) we're seeing and rating.

Still, you may be wondering about the abnormal gene studies or the brain malfunction theories of AD/HD. I will repeat here what others have said: *none* of the theories about what causes the symptoms we call AD/HD have proven to be true. For all of their searching, research scientists have not been able to find an abnormal gene, or brain malfunction, or any other disease or disorder that *can be viewed as a direct cause of* a thing called AD/HD.

What we *have* found is that even though some differences in genes or brains have been seen, we don't know yet what they mean. We still haven't found a "bad" gene that's responsible. And some studies show that it's the AD/HD medications, and *not* a thing called "AD/HD", that caused the brain shrinkage found in the brains of people diagnosed with AD/HD and medicated for it. We also know that many different things can create the same symptoms we call "AD/HD." Here are some examples:

- learning differences
- behavior management style
- stress or trauma
- poor nutrition or an unhealthy diet
- food and inhalant allergies or sensitivities
- hypoglycemia (low blood sugar)
- hyperthyroidism (overactive thyroid)
- severe hearing or vision problems

- sensitivities to chemicals like perfumes or cleaners
- metal or chemical poisoning in the body or brain from things like mercury, asbestos, lead, pesticides, or fertilizers

In the back of the book in Appendix A, I've included a chart that compares symptoms of "AD/HD" with symptoms we see in children experiencing a sensory integration dysfunction, learning-related visual problems, nutritional allergies, and average behavior for a child under age seven. You can see from the chart that each of these issues looks very much the same in children. Plus, the symptoms we call "AD/HD" overlap a lot with the symptoms used to diagnose more severe emotional issues like Conduct Disorder, Oppositional Defiant Disorder, Disruptive Behavior Disorder, Anxiety Disorder, Reactive Attachment Disorder, and Adjustment Disorder. In the end, the question we are still asking is "What *is* AD/HD?"

For years, part of making the official diagnosis of AD/HD was based on a person's response to the medication. If their behaviors "improved" as a result of the medication (in other words, if the child calmed down, focused better, got more done, was less sassy, etc.), it was assumed that the medicine was "working," which supported the belief that they must "have" AD/HD. In reality, *everyone* who takes the kinds of medications prescribed for AD/HD will have some kind of response to it.

There is evidence that if a person takes the medication and does not "have AD/HD," they will have the opposite response and become more active, energized, etc. This makes sense, because, after all, methylphenidate and the other drugs used to "treat" AD/HD are stimulants. This is why so many high school and college kids take it to have fun and help them stay awake and study longer when they are trying to "cram." This is also why some parents and professionals have risked their families and careers to steal their child's AD/HD drugs for personal and recreational use, and to have more energy to do what they needed to.

It is true that the drugs help people focus and get more done because they are stimulants that give people energy and affect the brain in a way that makes it focus differently. Plus, we must keep in mind that everyone's body system is somewhat unique because we are all exposed to different foods, toxins, experiences, etc. We can't expect every single person who takes a drug to have the same response to it. We may be able to say that "on average," people will respond a certain way, but in my opinion, even that is risky. So, how someone responds to the drugs is going to be a somewhat unique experience for them. And, there is still controversy about this among professionals who deal with it. We'll look more closely at these issues later in this chapter, in "How: Concerns About Drug Treatments for AD/HD" on page 24.

There was a time when I thought the AD/HD diagnosis might be helpful for children. That time has passed. Today, I believe that this label has done little more than create a system by which kids are too easily diagnosed and medicated for things that might best be dealt with differently. I also believe that AD/HD has become more about money and control than children's wellness:

- money – because the pharmaceutical companies are making a bundle off this diagnosis – more in this country than in all others;

- control – because people are looking for "quick fix" ways to "control" children's behavior.

What we've done as a nation is latched on to the AD/HD diagnosis and what is seen as the fastest and easiest solution: medication. Doctors are diagnosing children as young as two years old with AD/HD (and other disorders) and prescribing high-powered drugs to them. They do this even though there are no standards in place for diagnosing such young children, and the drugs they prescribe aren't approved for safety with children younger than six years of age. This adds up to a "double whammy" for kids. It's not only that doctors must make educated guesses about young children's behavior and what it means; it's that they squeeze kids into adult diagnoses, and then make more guesses about how the adult drugs will affect them, without really knowing the long-term impact of the drugs.

This is a very dangerous game we're playing with our children and their lives. It's like a crapshoot: you never know what the outcome will be, and it's always a risk. The sad fact is that this approach has created an entire generation of kids who are labeled and drugged, and whose future wellbeing is unknown. More than 7 million youngsters are on drugs for AD/HD. That's a lot of kids! Some of these kids are still in their developmental years, meaning that their bodies are still finishing their natural development. We know close to nothing about how these medications will affect their development in the future. For the more than 160 children who have already died from their AD/HD medication, they *lost* their future, and for what? Because we adults did not make the time to find healthy solutions that nourish their full potential. To me, this is a crime against kids.

This is no longer just a family concern. This has become an issue that relates to our whole society. If you care about your child (and all children), and you want to be well informed, and you are willing to explore all possibilities relating to your child's health, you will get something out of this book - even if you don't agree with all of it. In fact, I encourage you to question and do your own research on all things related to the wellbeing of your child. That's what I want each of us to do: question, study and talk about what we believe will be in the best service to our children, so that we can provide it for them. There's no harm in choosing to learn all we can about AD/HD so that we can make the best decisions possible when it comes to our children's wellbeing.

What: AD/HD From The Beginning

The first mention of behavior looking like today's "AD/HD" was made in 1902 by pediatrician George Still. He described "defects in moral control" and "volitional inhibition" in children. After the great flu epidemic of 1918, a lot of children who had been sick with brain infections like viral encephalitis and meningitis became impulsive, hyperactive, and inattentive. This pattern triggered research into the link between brain injuries and these symptoms. By the 1930s, the name "Minimal Brain Damage" was used to describe children with the symptoms.

In 1952, the American Psychiatric Association (APA) published the *Diagnostic and Statistical Manual of Mental Disorders* (DSM), a large book used to diagnose all known psychiatric disorders. This was the first time that being impulsive and hyperactive as a child became a disorder called "Hyperactivity of Childhood." When the APA updated the Manual in 1968 (DSM-II), "Hyperactivity of Childhood" was replaced with the diagnosis "Hyperkinetic Reaction of Childhood" to include hyperactivity, impulsivity, *and* wandering attention. By the time the third edition of the Manual was published in 1980 (DSM-III), the diagnosis was changed again to "Attention Deficit Disorder with or without Hyperactivity" (ADD/H). This was when the symptoms of inattention, impulsivity and hyperactivity became the basis of the disorder.

During the 1980s, it became clear that the kids didn't always show the behaviors linked to AD/HD in all places, under all conditions, and with all caregivers. Because of this, experts decided that the children's behavior was "rule-governed," or at least partly a response to what was expected of them in different places. Experts also saw that the kids diagnosed with hyperactivity were very different from the kids without it. Experts agreed that the behavior was affected by:

- how structured and demanding a setting was,
- the sex of the parent taking care of the child,
- what kinds of things the children were asked to do,
- how many times they were asked to do them,
- how new a situation was, and
- how soon and how often behavior was rewarded or punished

This led to another change in the name of the diagnosis when the DSM-III was revised in 1987, (DSM-IIIR). It became "Attention Deficit Hyperactivity Disorder" (ADHD).

As time passed, experts had trouble coming up with a clear way to define and measure the symptoms of ADHD. Studies using the DSM-IIIR criteria couldn't tell children diagnosed with ADHD apart from children without the diagnosis, or from children diagnosed with other mental disorders. So, in the fifth update of the Manual in 1994 (DSM-IV), the diagnosis was changed yet again to "Attention-Deficit/ Hyperactivity Disorder" (AD/HD) so that children could be diagnosed by which symptoms they showed the most.

In 2000, APA published an updated and corrected copy of the Manual, the DSM-IV-TR (*Diagnostic and Statistical Manual of Mental Disorders, Fourth Edition, Text Revision*), with the next revision (DSM-V) due out in May of 2012. Under AD/HD in the current revision, information was added to help doctors tell one type apart from the others. The four "types" as listed in the current Manual are:

Attention-Deficit/Hyperactivity Disorder, Predominantly Inattentive Type: show at least 6 symptoms of inattention for at least 6 months, and less than 6 symptoms of hyperactivity-impulsivity;

Attention-Deficit/Hyperactivity Disorder, Predominantly Hyperactive-Impulsive Type: show at least 6 symptoms of hyperactivity-impulsivity for at least 6 months, and less than 6 symptoms of inattention;

Attention-Deficit/Hyperactivity Disorder, Combined Type: show at least 6 symptoms from each area for at least 6 months;

Attention-Deficit/Hyperactivity Disorder, Not Otherwise Specified: when a child meets some, but not all, of the criteria for a diagnosis of AD/HD.

To diagnose AD/HD, some of the symptoms must be present before age 7, and it must be clear that the symptoms are causing "clinically significant impairment" (well above average problems for the person's age) in how they handle social settings, academics at school, or tasks at work. The symptoms must also be seen in at least two settings (e.g., home, school, work, community), and must not be linked to other diagnoses like a Pervasive Developmental Disorder, Schizophrenia, or to a Psychotic, Mood, Anxiety, Dissociate, or Personality Disorder.

The DSM-IV-TR warns against diagnosing AD/HD before elementary school age (6 years) since it's hard to tell the difference between average behaviors in active children and symptoms of AD/HD, and a lot of active toddlers don't go on to "develop" the disorder. It is also easier to notice and diagnose as kids are asked to stay focused for longer periods of time at school as they grow up. But this caution hasn't kept doctors and psychiatrists from diagnosing preschoolers with AD/HD and then prescribing drugs to them. In fact, research shows that from 1991 to 1995, the number of AD/HD drugs prescribed to children between the ages of 2 and 4 years doubled or tripled.

Controversy over the diagnosis of AD/HD

As the research on AD/HD grew, many professionals began to question whether or not AD/HD was truly a "disease." To address these concerns, the National Institutes of Health held a Consensus Conference in 1998, attended by professionals in the fields of psychology, psychiatry, medicine, education and health, to name a few. Their report concluded that "we do not have an independent, valid test for AD/HD, and there are no data to indicate that AD/HD is due to a brain malfunction." Yet the American Academy of Pediatrics (AAP) referred to it as a "disease or disorder" in the guidelines they created to help pediatricians make the diagnosis in 2000. Nearly ten years later, there is plenty of data to support the fact that it does not qualify as a "disease."

In his book, *Ritalin Is Not The Answer*, Dr. Stein reviews the four kinds of diseases:

1. infectious diseases, where a germ causes the symptoms,
2. contagious diseases, also where a germ causes the symptoms,
3. traumatic diseases, where there's some kind of harm to the body (like a blow to the head), and
4. systemic diseases, where the cells or chemicals of the body stop working right (as with cancer).

Some children who get brain or body sickness from infectious or contagious diseases end up with AD/HD-like symptoms, but most kids diagnosed with AD/HD today have never had a brain or body infection. We might also see the symptoms after a child has brain or body trauma or injury, but again, most kids diagnosed with AD/HD don't have this in their histories. So, we can count out diseases from germs and brain or body trauma as the cause of AD/HD; it is not caused by an infectious, contagious or traumatic disease.

But what about systemic diseases? Dr. Stein says that systemic diseases don't change much over time and don't increase as fast as AD/HD has without some kind of "dramatic, toxic change in the environment." Symptoms of systemic diseases also don't come and go depending on the setting and other external factors, as symptoms do with AD/HD. And, people certainly don't "outgrow" symptoms of systemic diseases.

Even if changes in the brain and the nervous system were found, this wouldn't prove that AD/HD is a disease because different things in the environment can create this kind of change. Dr. Stein explains that if changes in behavior and in the brain are caused by something in the environment, then it's called a "disorder," not a disease. If we called all changes caused by the environment a "disease," then everything we do or say would be a disease, which is absurd.

Dr. Stein reminds us that there are no tests that show an AD/HD "disease." The tests used to diagnose AD/HD don't measure failures in the brain or body; they only give us a way to see and log behavior.

So, what causes the symptoms we call AD/HD if not a "disease?" Can we say that AD/HD is a "disorder" rather than a disease or a medical condition? The DSM-IV-TR basically defines "mental disorder" as a behavioral, psychological, or biological "syndrome or pattern" that is notably different from what's considered the norm, and is creating physical distress, interfering with important areas of functioning, or is increasing the risk of harm or loss of freedom. It cannot be considered a typical response to an event (such as grief following a death).

Can we say then, that AD/HD is a "disorder?" Some say we can; others say we can't. There certainly is a profile of behaviors that have been attached to "AD/HD" that are viewed as outside the norm for kids; otherwise, it wouldn't be noticed at all. And although it would be hard to argue that the symptoms create "physical distress," it's clear that they can interfere with certain areas of functioning for kids. And you could argue that there is a risk of harm related to the impulsivity aspect of the diagnosis that could lead to a loss of freedom. It does not appear to be a typical response to an event, yet might it be a typical response to other factors in children's lives? This seems to be why there is so much debate over whether or not AD/HD is actually a "disorder" worth a diagnosis, especially when that diagnosis typically leads to risky drug treatments.

Instead of a "disease" or a "disorder," Dr. Stein thinks the symptoms we call AD/HD are found in children who:

1. are under-nurtured;
2. who don't have values like a love of learning, a willingness to work hard, long-term goals and delayed gratification (able to wait for "rewards");
3. who don't find value in school;
4. who don't get proper discipline; and
5. who are victims of class sizes that are just too big to manage with much success

These factors can certainly influence a child's functioning, and if extreme enough, can result in behavioral patterns that might be considered "atypical" or "abnormal." And there are many, many other things in a child's life that can create symptoms similar to those we call "AD/HD."

So, what causes AD/HD symptoms? Might they simply be a response to some other factors in a child's life? I believe that this is a question worth answering so that we can truly do what is in the best interest of our children around this issue.

Why: Questions About The Cause of AD/HD

Everything from studying brain structure with magnetic resonance imaging (MRI) scans, to studying brain metabolism with positron emission tomography (PET), to looking at brain blood flow and activity patterns through SPECT imaging, to studying genes through molecular biology, to looking at changes in the outside world has been done to find a cause of AD/HD. And you know what? In over 100 years of studying it, we still don't have one. Let's take a peek at some of the findings that this research has brought us.

Heredity. Although AD/HD symptoms do tend to "run in families," so far no gene has been found that definitively links it to heredity. Considering that family members living together are exposed to the same external influences (like food, toxins and stressors), it is hard to say that AD/HD symptoms in multiple family members are due to heredity and not to their exposure to one of these other factors. And, *everyone* has a 50-50 chance of being diagnosed just by being born. To look at the issue of heredity further, studies were done with identical twins. If a gene were truly responsible for the symptoms, you'd expect that both identical twins – two people with identical genes – would have the symptoms and be diagnosed. But these studies show that both identical twins don't always have AD/HD symptoms and are not always diagnosed with AD/HD.

"Broken Brain." In the beginning, experts noticed a link between the symptoms of AD/HD and some type of brain injury or insult. Today, we've found that even though children who've had birth or head traumas or brain infections *do* tend to show the symptoms, most kids diagnosed with AD/HD *don't* have these things in their histories. When studying the brain itself with things like MRI or PET scans and neurotransmitter activity, experts do not know what causes the differences they see. Although it is true that the brains of people diagnosed with AD/HD are smaller in size and don't operate in the same ways as people who don't have the diagnosis, scientists agree that the brain changes could be due to the use of drugs prescribed to "treat" their AD/HD, and not to what we call "AD/HD." Others admit that the differences could be linked to things like stress, parenting style, classroom structure, toxins or any number of other external factors that haven't been ruled out yet. The bottom line is that we have not found a direct link between what we call AD/HD and a "broken brain."

Nutrition. Most people agree that the American diet is far less nutritious today than it has ever been before, leaving kids without the essential nutrients their bodies need to work right. Not only have we become a "fast food nation," but the food we buy in grocery stores is less nutritious and more toxic than ever before because of (1) depletion of nutrients in the soil, (2) the use of toxic chemicals during growing and (3) the use of toxic packaging materials. Americans also eat way too much processed foods and sugar, which create any number of health problems in the body. Together, these things can overload the body's natural defense systems for handling toxins from the outside world and leave it open to developing sensitivities to foods or airborne allergens like pollen or dust. The body and brain's response to these things can look like the symptoms we call "AD/HD."

Many experts believe that what we call "AD/HD" is caused by eating foods that are nutritionally empty or even toxic. Poor nutrition and weakened bodies cause things like allergies or sensitivities, thyroid dysfunction, heavy metal imbalances, fatty acid deficiencies, vitamin or mineral deficiencies, yeast overgrowth, or "leaky gut syndrome" (in which the digestive tract doesn't work right). Research does show that these things are a part of many, but not all, cases of what we diagnose as AD/HD.

Technology. We are living in the "Technological Age," in which new technologies are made available every day. Today's kids have grown up within this technological boom, and have been exposed to – from birth – a much higher and faster level of stimulation in their everyday worlds than any generation before them. They have computers that run at "high speeds;" cell phones that allow instant communication from wherever they are and can even take pictures, send and receive emails, and watch and make videos; electronic, palm-sized calendars, planners, stereos and games; fax machines; microwave ovens; digital cameras; and any number of other gadgets at their disposal. All of these technologies allow us to do more and more things in faster and faster ways.

Some experts believe that since all of these things push the limits of our senses, kids have grown up with a "heightened sensory awareness." Now, their bodies and brains are trained to deal with high levels of intense, fast-paced sensory stimulation in one of two ways: either the body goes into symptoms of anxiety, acting out, impatience, intolerance, inattention and agitation when that level of stimulation is not available, or the body goes into overwhelm and responds with symptoms like withdrawal, desensitization, depersonalization and emotional separation.

Some argue that the symptoms we call "AD/HD" are really the brain's attempts to adjust to the different kinds of stimulation it's being exposed to in today's high-tech world. Logically, this makes sense; however, there is not yet enough research to say that today's technology is responsible for all the symptoms kids are showing us, at least, not all by itself.

Does AD/HD Exist as a Unique "Disorder?"

There is still a lot of controversy around the AD/HD diagnosis, and many experts share the concern that what we call "AD/HD" is really normal differences in behavior that either stay within normal ranges or move into extremes based on a person's relationship with their environment. What most experts do agree on is that more than one thing is probably responsible for the symptoms we call "AD/HD." They also agree that a lot of people diagnosed with AD/HD are actually dealing with other medical or mental health conditions.

The symptoms of inattention, restlessness, impulsivity, and social or school struggles (the most common things seen as AD/HD) can be a part of many other concerns, including insomnia (trouble sleeping), substance use and abuse, learning differences, severe problems within the hearing or visual systems, child abuse or neglect, depression, severe stress or trauma, sensory integration weaknesses, head injuries, diabetes hypoglycemia (too little sugar in the blood), thyroid problems, nutritional imbalances, allergies and sensitivities, and too much metal in the body (like silver, mercury, or lead). Because of this, it's hard to know if the behaviors a child is showing are due to some disorder called "AD/HD" or to something else going on in their lives that hasn't been identified, or to a combination of things. The typical assessments used to diagnose "AD/HD" aren't sufficient to rule out all the other factors that can create similar symptoms.

So my question is: "Is it fair, is it smart, is it healthy, is it responsible, and is it loving of us as a society to treat our children for something we're not even certain exists, particularly with drugs that alter their brains and bodies?" Today, the typical treatment program for AD/HD is a schedule of drugs, and if a kid's lucky, maybe some therapy or behavioral interventions as well. The concern that many professionals share is that drugs are meant to be a "last line" of treatment, not the first line of treatment that they've become, particularly when dealing with developing children.

Unfortunately, major medical groups such as the American Association of Pediatrics support the use of drugs as a first line of treatment for AD/HD, although major psychological groups such as the National Association of School Psychologists do not support this. However, since it is the doctors and psychiatrists that prescribe the drugs, things probably won't change much until the medical and psychiatric leadership associations shift their views and guidelines.

So, what are the concerns about drug treatments for "AD/HD" of so many professionals who work with children?

How: Concerns About Drug Treatments For AD/HD

To be sure, prescription drugs have found their place in the treatment of AD/HD and other symptoms experienced by children in this country. In fact, the U.S. Drug Enforcement Agency reports that between 1990 and 1997, the production of methylphenidate (commonly known as "Ritalin") grew by 700%, with 90% of that being used in this country alone. Today we know that at least 7 million kids in America are taking some kind of prescription drug for a diagnosis of AD/HD.

How someone responds to the drugs is part of how doctors make the diagnosis: a positive response is viewed as evidence that a person has AD/HD. This is based on the belief of some experts that the drugs only have a positive effect on people who have the disorder. However, based on an extensive review of the research, the American Academy of Child and Adolescent Psychiatry concluded in 2002 that the drugs improve behavior and attention in *everyone*, not just those with symptoms of AD/HD. So, in my opinion, it is not good practice to use positive response to the drugs as a way of affirming a diagnosis of AD/HD.

Many experts are very concerned about the increase in drug prescriptions to children younger than 5 years old because there are no studies that tell us about the safety or effectiveness of the drugs for this age group. Experts also question the practice of using the current guidelines (which are based almost exclusively on studies with people age 6 to adult) to diagnose very young children with AD/HD, especially since this usually leads to a drug prescription. The drugs have a disruptive effect on children's body and brain development, and we don't know all of the long-term effects they have on their overall health and wellbeing.

There is also a concern about over-prescription of drugs for AD/HD, and of possible links to drug abuse. In fact, the U.S. has the highest rates of methylphenidate (or Ritalin) use in the world. The International Narcotics Control Board (INCB), which monitors global drug addiction and abuse, noted that methylphenidate is one of the top ten controlled substances that is stolen, used and abused. The INCB is also concerned by the fact that children in the U.S. tend to take the drugs for longer periods of time than children in other countries. The fact is that millions of high school and college students in the U.S. admit to abusing

18

the drug, thinking of it as "legal speed." And there are also a number of stories out there from parents and professionals who stole and got addicted to their child's methylphenidate prescriptions.

It is important to remember that all the drugs really do is create a "drugged state" within children so that they appear calmer and more mentally focused for as long as the drug is in their system. This state disappears as soon as the drug's effects wear off, not because children's symptoms are so severe, but because they are no longer under the influence of these mind-altering drugs. Tolerance can develop with some people, so that stronger doses are needed to get the same results. Not only do the symptoms reappear without the drug, but they also tend to be more severe. Many people experience "withdrawal" when the drug is stopped, and act out behaviorally or for some, become suicidal. And they can be psychologically (if not physically) addicting. The verdict is still out as to whether or not the drugs are "gateways" to future drug use and abuse.

The truth is that today, although 60% to 80% of the children who take stimulant drugs do get some *short-term* relief from their symptoms, research clearly shows that there are no lasting effects to justify the many health risks involved, especially for preschoolers. And there are so many health risks linked to the drugs prescribed for AD/HD. These range from weight loss, headaches, stomach aches and stunted growth to permanent damage to the heart, liver and kidneys, to death for some.

The chart below summarizes common and uncommon side effects of the drugs:

Common, more mild side effects	Possible severe side effects
Stomachaches	Bone marrow suppression
Headaches	Seizures
Loss of appetite	Parkinson's Disease
Moodiness	Chromosomal damage (early findings)
Sleep problems	Changes in brain size
Stunted growth	Psychosis
Edginess	Liver or Kidney toxicity or poisoning
Over-focusing	Liver problems or failure
Tics/Tourette's Syndrome	Liver cancer
Rebound behaviors	Heart problems or failure
	Death

The problem is that the drug review process used by the FDA is not sufficient to ensure that all possible harmful effects of a new drug are known before it is allowed into the market. Plus, it would be impossible for the FDA to know how every drug would interact with each individual's body.

To date, at least 160 children have died as a direct result of using methylphenidate or another drug commonly prescribed for AD/HD, sometimes in combination with other psychoactive drugs. There are very recent cases of other types of drugs being pulled from the market for their role in fewer deaths than that (Remember the quick weight loss drugs, "Ephedra" and "Fen-Phen?"). To date, a couple of the drugs used to treat "AD/HD" have been pulled from the market due to their serious risks, first in other countries and later in the U.S., for example, Cylert and Adderall.

So why are so many of these AD/HD drugs still on the market and so widely accepted and used by doctors? There are several possible reasons for this. What I will share here is that people see "quick results" or changes in children who take the drugs. Drugs are fast-acting agents on the body. They move quickly into children's systems and have a powerful effect on their brains, which then triggers reactions in the rest of the body. It feels like an easy solution to dealing with kid's behaviors that doesn't take much effort from adults. It is easy to hand kids a pill. And doctors tell parents that the drugs are safe and effective, so why not?

Money is also a factor. There is a lot of money involved in the sale of drugs used to treat "AD/HD." The drug companies are making a bundle! It's important for you to know that most of the research done on the safety of the drugs is funded by the drug companies themselves. In recent years, it has come to light that these companies haven't always been completely truthful in their public reports about the risks and safety of their drugs.

The reality is that it takes years before the long-term effects of a drug can truly be known; often, the full truth about the health risks of a drug do not surface until years after it has been on the market. This is true for other drugs as well, not just AD/HD drugs; it's the nature of the process. People have to take a new drug for say, ten years, for us to really know how it will affect the body to be on that particular drug for that length of time. So, essentially, people are guinea pigs for long-term risks of prescription drugs. All doctors can really tell parents about a drug is what the research has shown, which generally means that a new drug has been shown to be "safe" under certain conditions in the short term, *not* the long term. This is the information the FDA bases its decision on when deciding whether or not a drug is safe to release to the public.

Instead of spending our time and energy on that can of worms, however, we turn our attention to the main reason for this book: to introduce you to a new model of children's health care and to expose you to trustworthy and healthy options for dealing with your child's behaviors that don't involve drugs. For those of you who are interested in a detailed discussion of the possible causes of AD/HD, the legitimacy of the diagnosis, the pluses and minuses of using drugs as "treatment," and why the AD/HD diagnosis persists, I refer you to the *AD/HD Generation Companion Book*.

2

A Holistic Model of Wellness For Children

The Value of Shifting Our Approach

EACH OF US has our own idea about what it means to be "healthy." I would argue that being truly healthy means experiencing the vitality, vigor, strength, and life force of body, mind, emotions, spirit and energy. I believe that when one of these areas of our being is out of balance or in disharmony with the rest, we experience a state of discomfort or "dis-ease" (either physical, mental, emotional, spiritual, and/or energetic). The goal is to keep all the parts of ourselves working up to their potential and in harmony with the whole. This is no easy task! I believe that it takes motivation, discipline, and will. You must be motivated to want to be as healthy as you can be. You must be disciplined to do what it takes to achieve health, and you must be willing to work at maintaining your health. Simply having the intention to be healthy and respecting yourself enough to take responsibility and try your best each day can create important changes in your health and in your life.

To view "health" as each part of ourselves working in harmony to create a healthy state of being, means to view health from a holistic perspective. Each part of ourselves and our lives combine in a unique way to make a whole, integrated package that becomes "us." The holistic model of wellness addresses the physical, mental, emotional, spiritual, and energetic parts of our health. The focus of a holistic approach is treating the body as a complete working system instead of a bunch of separate parts. A holistic health model says that dis-ease in any one of these parts throws the whole system out of balance, while health in each of these parts will lead to health in the whole system.

People in the field of holistic health care believe that focusing on the active prevention of dis-ease and viewing the body as a whole system working within a certain context is a more positive, effective and efficient way to manage health care than randomly treating a person's symptoms. In other words, holistic health care focuses on balancing each person's life systems rather than bandaging individual symptoms. This way, the "root" of a symptom can be found and life changes can be made to make it less likely that such a symptom will return.

Naturopathic doctors (NDs) are licensed physicians who practice a holistic health model. They respect people's ability to heal themselves and consider their patients active partners in creating their own wellness. In fact, individuality and responsibility are central to a holistic approach. This model of health care – seeing each person as primarily responsible for their wellbeing in partnership with a professional -- has been a successful part of some Eastern medicine approaches for thousands of years. Two examples are traditional Ayurvedic medicine originating in India, and traditional Chinese medicine. Both are time-tested, whole systems of wellness that involve self-care of the physical, mental, emotional, spiritual, and/or energetic bodies in order to maintain good health and prevent disease.

Naturopathic medicine follows a holistic health model. Naturopathic doctors emphasize things like nutrition, herbal and homeopathic remedies, exercise and acupuncture. Their focus is on prevention. They are trained in the medical sciences and emergency procedures, just as allopathic doctors are (those with a modern Western approach to wellness). Although they are trained in modern diagnostic equipment and techniques, they also rely on the body to "tell," or signal, them as to what is happening internally.

This is different from allopathic medicine, which usually follows a "doctor as expert" model, in which patients defer a great deal of responsibility for their wellness to their doctors. Allopathic doctors tend to focus on treatment of symptoms rather than on prevention, and generally rely on prescription drugs and surgery to deal with most health issues. This approach can be helpful in a crisis, since drugs and surgery are "fast-acting" on the body. But for most other health issues, a holistic approach provides an effective, less intrusive and more long-term choice for creating wellness.

Many people cling to the false belief that they can live their lives in whatever way they want, and that when something "goes wrong," or they start having uncomfortable symptoms, their doctor can make them well again. But chances are that unless the patient takes some personal responsibility for their health by making lifestyle changes, their symptoms probably will not *stay* gone for long, or new ones will show up. That is why a holistic approach might involve a balancing of things like diet, exercise, body awareness, changes in behavior, and personal responsibility within the environment that sustains you. While there is no denying that there are times when swift medical or surgical action is needed, the emphasis of a holistic approach is on educating patients so they can be in control of their own health (and avoid a dependence on doctors, drugs and surgery).

The World Health Organization (WHO) defines health as "...more than simply the absence of illness. It is the *active* state of physical, emotional, mental, and social well-being." This definition is aligned with the holistic approach to health which says that we can create our wellness through the lifestyle we choose, including: 1) how we take care of ourselves (e.g., diet and exercise habits, substance use, rest and relaxation habits); 2) what we do to the environment that sustains us (e.g., managing pollutants and toxins); and 3) how we behave (e.g., living with integrity and respect). So, maintaining health means taking active steps to stay physically and emotionally fit, spiritually and energetically strong, mentally stable, and socially and behaviorally responsible. When we experience a state of dis-ease in any of these areas, we are probably ignoring our relationship to some part of our whole system of being. This creates an imbalance not only within ourselves but also in how we relate to the world around us. A holistic approach supports us in finding and keeping balance among all of the areas of our wellbeing, so that we can function at our highest potential.

Children's ability to function at their best is linked to their state of health in each of these areas, just as yours is. Parents are responsible for teaching children about living a healthy lifestyle, which includes their physical, mental, social-emotional, spiritual, and energetic health. This holistic view means that you commit to thinking more in terms of prevention than treatment. You become mindful of what goes into your child's body, not only through their mouth, but through their other sensory organs as well. Are they exposed to cigarette smoke, alcohol, or drugs? Toxic chemicals, noise pollution, or too much sun? What kind of food and drinks do they nourish themselves with? Do they rest, sleep, and exercise enough? Do they drink enough water? Do they read, listen to, or watch things that feed their spirit or things that contain heavy energy (violence, cruelty, crudeness, vulgarity, porn, etc.)? Attending to all of these things is a part of managing your child's overall health in a preventative and holistic manner. Keeping your child in a strong state of physical, mental, social-emotional, spiritual, and energetic health means that they will be better prepared to be their best every day.

A Holistic Health Care Approach for Symptoms of AD/HD

With all the medication scares today, many parents are wondering if there are safe and effective ways to address children's behavioral symptoms, such as those that are linked to the AD/HD diagnosis, without the use of medications. The answer to this question is that yes, there are many ways to address these symptoms. What parents need to know, however, is that there is not one, "sure-fire" treatment that works for all people with symptoms like inattention, hyperactivity, or impulsivity. Instead, different people respond to different interventions. Research shows that the uniqueness of a person's situation dictates what treatment(s) may work best for them. This idea - that each person must be viewed as unique, and must be treated within the context of their environment - is part of what holistic health care is all about. That is why I believe that there is a positive match between a holistic health care approach and treating the symptoms of AD/HD.

We've already reviewed some of the reasons that I support revisiting our approach to AD/HD. In a nutshell, instead of mass-diagnosing and drugging our kids, I believe we should rely primarily on a holistic approach that views each child and their symptoms as unique. I find it curious and of concern that the US has the highest rate of diagnosing (and drugging) for AD/HD in the world, a rate that's higher than most other countries combined. Why is that? Could it be as simple a difference as our approach to children's wellbeing?

Since so many questions remain unanswered about the AD/HD diagnosis and the drugs prescribed to children because of it, I believe we have a responsibility to our children to shift our approach away from the medical model (relying on drugs and surgery) and towards a holistic model (relying on preventive and natural supports). Along with that, I believe that it simply makes sense to use a health care model that *starts* with the safest and most gentle remedies and *only* moves up the scale to the less safe and less gentle remedies if needed. Logically, this makes sense. If I had a headache, for example, I would be foolish to start my search for pain relief by having brain surgery, instead of trying other, more mild types of pain relief first. Ethically, it also makes sense as a society to choose safe, gentle treatments for children's symptoms before trying things that could have serious long-term effects on their growth and development.

Holistic health care takes into account the various parts of a person and their life - their history, the environments they live in, their character and how they behave, their experiences, and the status of their physical, mental, social-emotional, and spiritual/energetic beings - that contribute to their state of wellness. It also focuses on prevention and includes personal responsibility for maintaining health and wellbeing. Treatments are chosen to match each person's profile of balance and imbalance within their whole being and in their environment. These include many different approaches, depending on a person's needs. Again, one key to holistic health care is viewing each situation as unique, rather than assuming that similar symptom patterns are rooted in the same cause and will respond to the same treatment for everyone.

Naturopathy and AD/HD

Naturopathy is a model of treatment that stresses the use of physical methods (such as massage) and natural substances (such as herbs) to promote wellness, and avoids reliance on harsh drugs and surgery. In my view, naturopathic approaches to good health are at the mild end of the scale of treatment choices, while prescription drugs are at the more severe end. Let us remember that research supports the use of drugs as a *last resort* for treating the symptoms of AD/HD, rather than as the first line of treatment that it has become – especially with children younger than six years of age.

There are many professionals working with children who, like myself, believe that choosing a more natural approach to the treatment of symptoms such as inattention, hyperactivity and impulsivity is more acceptable than the use of powerful drugs. For example, Drs. Tom Cushman and Thomas Johnson recently wrote a three-part series of articles on managing attentional problems in children. The series was published in *Communiqué*, the professional newspaper of the National Association of School Psychologists. These clinicians believe that problems such as inattention are best addressed using a holistic model and a comprehensive treatment approach. For instance, they suggest that parents, caring adults and children:

1. spend more time together;
2. spend more time in nature, away from technological stimuli;
3. learn the importance of good sleeping habits, good nutrition, regular exercise, relaxation, and supportive relationships;
4. allow verbal, musical, or artistic expression of emotions; and
5. allow time for physical movement at school.

Working with naturopathy means opening your mind to a new way of thinking about health and wellbeing. Many of the healing approaches in naturopathy do not lend themselves to the standard method of research supported in Western medicine - the "double-blind" research study. As Dr. Mary Ann Bloch explained in her book, *No More Ritalin*, "To do a double-blind study, one must be able to do something to the patient that can be kept secret from the patient and from the doctor. There are not many treatments other than drugs that can work in a double-blind format, but scientists...believe that this method is the only way to substantiate anything useful in medicine. If the method of treatment has not been through a double-blind study, the method is not acceptable in Western allopathic medicine. This is true even with treatments such as acupuncture, herbs, and homeopathy - treatments that have been used successfully for thousands of years in other parts of the world."[1]

What we need to remember about health is that it involves all the systems of the body, including the physical, mental, emotional and spiritual/energetic. Healing these systems goes beyond the physical and into the ethereal (non-material, energetic) realm. Since we know that everything, including our bodies, is made up of nothing more than space, light, and energy that vibrates or resonates at a certain frequency, we can use this energy for healing purposes. By everything, I mean *everything* - stones, tables, trees, people, animals, cells, bacteria, parasites, insects, fish, birds, desks, food...*everything*.

Our physical senses (taste, smell, touch, sound, sight) are generally too weak to pick up on these energies without mechanical help. There are some people, however, who have cleared out and opened up the systems of their body enough to be able to "sense" these energies, and can even "read" them, where the average, "clogged-up" person cannot. We generally call them psychics, and say that they have "extrasensory perception" (or ESP), meaning that they can perceive things that reside beyond or outside of what the ordinary senses can detect.

Dr. Kevin Ross Emery is one of those people. He has a Bachelor of Arts degree in Business and Psychology from the University of New Hampshire, and both a Maters and Doctorate degree in Divinity from the Universal Brotherhood University. He is the founder of Synergy Business Consulting™ and co-creator and teacher of the Wei Chi Tibetan Reike™ system of natural healing. He is author and coauthor of several books and tapes, including his most recent, *Managing The Gift: Alternative Approaches For Attention Deficit Disorder*. Although he has been a spiritual coach and counselor in New Hampshire since the early 1990s, his current focus is on alternative approaches for dealing with AD/HD.

Dr. Emery does what he calls 'medical intuitive scans'. He describes each person as having one body system with four levels of being. He explains that when he scans a person, he gets information about their physical, emotional, mental and spiritual/energetic levels of being. From this scan, he receives information about where their system is out of balance, and what needs to happen to correct it.

When the systems of our bodies get out of balance, the energy patterns generated by the body shift. Healing, therefore, can include work that is done to balance out the energy patterns once again. This type of healing, which Drs. Reichenberg-Ullman and Ullman refer to as 'energy medicine' in their book, *Ritalin Free Kids*, is what is accessed in such time-tested therapies as acupuncture, acupressure, kinesiology, homeopathy, flower remedies, aromatherapy, Reiki, CranioSacral therapy and massage. Many of these approaches are reviewed in Part Two of this book. As Drs. Reichenberg-Ullman and Ullman explain, energy medicine does not necessarily work on a biochemical level, and we may not "fully understand how to measure, analyze, or evaluate" it, but it is clinically effective, nonetheless.

A Model of Support Without Drugs

In his book, *Ritalin is not the answer*, Dr. David Stein, a Clinical Psychologist and Associate Professor of Psychology in Virginia, writes that he has identified a treatment program for changing children's behavioral, thinking and motivational patterns that gets rid of the need for drugs for those diagnosed with AD/HD. He has developed what he calls "The Caregivers' Skills Program" which consists of five key points:

1. Children must be taken off their prescription drugs for the symptoms of AD/HD. Dr. Stein believes that drugs like Ritalin mask the behaviors that are targeted for change. He maintains that if we are to successfully change children's way of thinking and behaving, old patterns must be present so that they can be replaced with new ones when they occur. Dr. Stein believes that only in this way do children gain an awareness of their patterns and learn to control them, and only in this way will they truly change.

2. Children's "AD/HD" is not due to a disease or medical condition.
As we reviewed earlier in this book, AD/HD does not meet criteria as
a disease, and it is not considered a medical condition. Dr. Stein believes that children with this label are "normal," yet have learned inappropriate behaviors and faulty thinking. He also believes that they
lack the motivation to learn and to perform well in school, and lack
positive values. Dr. Stein believes that the best way to address what
we call AD/HD is to use therapeutic techniques to teach and support
the changes you want your child to make. He proposes renaming
the AD/HD patterns as "inattentive" (IA) and "highly misbehaving"
(HM) children to account for the lack of a medical disease.

**3. Children must be taught new ways of thinking as well as behav-
ing.** Dr. Stein sees IA and HM children as those who engage in "not
thinking." He maintains that these children need to be taught how to
think for themselves and how to monitor their own behavior, rather
than relying on others to think for them and control their behavior.

4. Change must begin at home. Dr. Stein views parenting as a major
component in the change process. He suggests that unless children
learn to manage their own thinking and behavior at home, school
performance will continue to suffer. In his experience, once home patterns improve, changing school patterns becomes "relatively easy."

5. Use a comprehensive approach to change. In The Caregivers'
Skills Program, Dr. Stein focuses on teaching parents what is producing their child's IA or HM patterns, and how to correct them. The
program includes "every behavioral and motivational problem" that
affects the child's success at home and school. Dr. Stein believes that
this is necessary to effectively create change.

Dr. Stein's Program strongly supports a non-drug, holistic approach to addressing children's behaviors. It is also aligned with
many of the ideas you will read in the following chapters of this
book. So let's take a closer look at several holistic options you can use
to nurture children's development and vitality.

About Part Two

The goal of Part Two is to provide you with safe, gentle, natural and holistic ways to support the workings of your child's whole body, so they can stay successful, healthy and disease free in both the short and the long term. *My decision to include certain methods or products in this book does not mean that I endorse them or their use with children, just as the exclusion of certain methods or products does not mean that they should not be used.* I simply offer a discussion about some of the more popular holistic approaches that are available to you, should you choose to explore them further.

Keep in mind that the body works as a total package including the systems of the physical body, the mind, the emotions, the spirit, and the energetic Being. When any one of these systems is out of balance, signs of "distress" will show up. This "warning" plan is wired into our body's operating software. It is there to tell us when one of the systems is in need of some extra time and attention. It is similar to your car making a funny noise or smell when something is wrong with a part of its mechanisms. As adults, we need to support children in keeping their bodies and all of its systems healthy and working properly, so that they can show up ready to be their best every day.

The information contained in Part Two certainly does not cover every possibility, but it does touch on some of the most used and discussed methods in terms of holistic health care. The fact that I do not cover each area equally does not mean that I support one method over any other. My goal is to alert you to the many choices available for nurturing children's wholeness without the use of pharmaceutical drugs. *Self-treatment is not recommended or advised, due to the uniqueness of each individual and the complexities involved with holistic healing. Consult a professional holistic health care provider before trying any of the remedies mentioned.* I have included a reference guide with lists of resources for more information, should you choose to explore an area further.

PART TWO

Holistic Ways to Support Children

3

PARENTING

Fine-tuning the parent-child relationship for positive change

Introduction

You MIGHT BE amazed at the difference that a few shifts in your parenting – how you relate to your child – can make in your relationship with them. Part of your child's behavior is driven by how they perceive what's happening around them, how each situation makes them feel, and how they feel able (or not) to interact with it. By becoming more aware of the signals you're giving to your child, you can gain a certain amount of control over their responses to you. There are some tools that you can use to make it easier for your child to respond in a positive way to your signals.

This chapter includes information about the art of parenting so that you can fine-tune your parenting skills. You will read about how parenting styles, attitudes, behaviors, beliefs and expectations influence children's behavior. You will also learn some new strategies to support more positive and effective communication between you and your children. Problem solving is also covered, with special attention given to understanding and identifying the goals of children's behavior. In general, I provide a "snapshot" of some of my favorite parenting strategies from the field of psychology.

At the end of the chapter, I provide eight hints for getting things done with challenging children. *Keep in mind that whenever you change the way you relate to your child, their behavior may get worse before getting better. If you stick it out and consistently use a new strategy for two weeks, you should see positive change by the end of that time.* Don't give up or in too soon. Making changes in your parenting takes practice, patience and persistence.

In my view, of all the parenting books on the market, one of the most useful is the original, *Systematic Training for Effective Parenting (STEP): The Parent's Handbook,* by Don Dinkmeyer & Gary McKay. Today, the *STEP* program has grown into a series of parenting handbooks for children at specific age groups, so you can select the one that best fits your needs. Most other parenting programs that I have studied include the same, or very similar, principles as those covered by Don and Gary, and their books are very "user friendly." Many of the ideas I review in this chapter are based on their work (Why reinvent the wheel?). They don't belong in any specific order; they are simply areas of parenting to be visited and considered. Supporting children's behaviors through parenting strategies fits with a holistic health care model because it promotes wellness through prevention. Let's look at nine key areas of parenting that can be fine-tuned for positive change.

One: Parenting Style

One of the first steps toward encouraging a more harmonious relationship with your children is to examine your parenting style. Parenting style plays a large part in children's behavior patterns. For example, we know that self-confident, successful children come from homes that have a loving environment where parents respect them, show an interest in them, and let them know they are proud of them. These parents are also less permissive and use a democratic style of decision-making in which children's views are valued.

There are generally three styles of parenting: authoritarian, permissive, and authoritative. We know that an authoritarian style, in which parents are "the boss" and children are expected to blindly do as they are told, leaves children feeling incompetent and incapable of making decisions. They do not trust their own judgment, and are often afraid of making a mistake. They may feel that their opinion does not matter, and that they have little worth in the family or the world. Some children become rebellious around this style, and do everything they are told not to do. They become argumentative and show an "I don't care" attitude. They may break rules simply because they can.

In contrast, a permissive parenting style in which parents allow children to do whatever they want, or give in to a child's demands, does not teach them to respect personal and other boundaries. They lack a sense of responsibility for their behavior and will blame others instead. Children raised in this way tend to push the limits of rules. They generally feel that they have a right to do what they want. They tend to disregard the feelings of others. Often, their attitude is, "My way or no way." They may tantrum or become angry or aggressive when they cannot have their way. They think if they keep trying, adults will eventually give in and they will get their way. So, they keep trying.

Finally, an authoritative style in which parents give limited choices, teaches children to take responsibility for their behavior and accept consequences. Children from authoritative homes tend to be more confident and successful. They understand, accept, and respect limits. They generally trust their own judgment and are better able to make successful choices. They are more sensitive to the feelings and rights of others, and are more willing to compromise and cooperate. They may ask, "What will happen if…?" and learn to evaluate their choices before taking action.

Knowing the type of parenting style you rely on the most with your children may help you understand some of their behaviors. Then, you can decide what parts, if any, of your style you would like to revisit and shift to better suit your long-term goals with your child.

Two: Parenting Attitudes and Behaviors

It is a well-known fact that people influence each other. One person's attitudes and behaviors will affect those around them. This is especially true with close, personal relationships, such as that between parent and child. So, a second area of parenting to examine is how your attitudes and behaviors affect your children's behavior. In this section, I review two relatively new views of parenting attitudes and behaviors that help to explain and resolve tense parent-child interactions.

Dr. Bryan Post's Family-Centered Regulatory Parenting Approach: Dr. Post is a Licensed Clinical Social Worker with a private practice in Oklahoma. He uses a stress model of children's behavior that I will summarize here so you can understand his parenting approach described in this section.

Based on Dr. Post's Stress Model, we can consider that children who have experienced traumatic events or circumstances while in the uterus or during their first seven years of life probably have three differences in their brain:

1. an underdeveloped hippocampus (the thinking part of the brain that manages our emotions);

2. a dysfunctional orbital-frontal cortex (the center of our social and emotional functioning); and

3. an overzealous amygdala (the threat receptor in the brain that tells us if we need to go into "fight, flight or freeze" mode).

As a result, communication between their amygdala and their hippocampal/orbito-frontal cortex gets distorted. Chronically stressed children tend to misread most events in their environment as threats even when they are not, and respond to them from a place of fear. In other words, they tend to go into "fight, flight or freeze" mode when they don't need to. This is the first piece of the puzzle.

The second piece of this puzzle is that most of what we communicate to others is conveyed through our behavior, not our words. In fact, 90% of our communication is nonverbal, done with gestures and expressions instead of words. The brain receives the most stimulation from eye contact and touch. Children pick up on these nonverbal messages. They can feel when a caregiver is distressed, and this triggers their amygdala. For children whose hippocampus and/or orbital-frontal cortex is underdeveloped or damaged, this shakes their sense of security and their ability to stay regulated. Like adults, children communicate through their behavior, so distressed children "act out" their emotions. This is how they communicate the stress they are feeling both internally, and externally in the family.

This means that the best way for caregivers to help children when they are "acting out" (dysregulated) is to stay regulated themselves. Then, they can support children in returning to a state of regulation when they are emotionally distressed. Oftentimes, what we do instead is react emotionally, which fuels the child's own distress. Or, we medicate them, which can make it harder for them to communicate what they are really feeling inside and outside of themselves. Drugs also create a mask that covers up the root cause of the behavior so parents and caregivers have a harder time figuring out how to soothe them.

The goals of Dr. Post's approach to managing children's behaviors are basically to:

1.   provide a safe and calm environment that will allow the child to begin to return to a state of regulation;

2.   switch off their overactive amygdala; and

3.   help them become aware of their true feelings so that regulation can occur.

When children are allowed to release the stress they are feeling, the rational part of their brain (their hippocampus) turns on again. This puts them in the position of being ready to see their surroundings more accurately and for caregivers to teach them more appropriate responses.

Dr. Post says that caregivers "must be willing to be response-able" for children. This means that they must be willing to do their own healing so that they can work at staying regulated themselves, which then allows them to provide the kind of environment children need to do the same. In this way, Dr. Post's priority is working with caregivers first, followed by the family system and the caregiver-child relationship once the parents are ready.

The parents' task is to create a calm environment so that the child can return to a state of regulation. This involves a three-phase intervention strategy in which caregivers (1) reflect on their own feelings; (2) relate their feelings to the child, and show understanding by asking them to voice theirs; and (3) safely release the feelings, which allows the environment to shift and the child to return to a state of regulation. This three-phase process helps to calm the stress, gives the hippocampus (rational part of the brain) a chance to turn on, and creates the kind of environment that the orbito-frontal cortex (the center of social-emotional functioning) needs to complete its development and start working like it's supposed to. Dr. Post reminds parents to approach children at their emotional age rather than their cognitive age. This is because their levels of development in each of these areas can be different.

Although this is a simplified version of Dr. Post's stress model, I think it gives you an idea of how it works. There are many other parenting strategies that can be used to deal with children's challenging behaviors, but I encourage you to keep Dr. Post's model in mind as you read, because some of these other strategies won't work well with children who fit into his stress model. For example, children who have been exposed to high amounts of stress in their lives, and are likely in a chronic state of dysregulation, will not respond to traditional parenting or discipline techniques. These children act out on a daily basis. They are not equipped – from a neurophysiological standpoint – to make the right decisions or choices. They are too stressed internally, which controls how they respond to the events and people around them. Dr. Post says that "when we give consequences to these children… we are not identifying their emotions or their stress; we are ignoring the root of the problem, and almost punishing them for something that they do not have any control over."[2]

Dr. Post believes that traditional behavioral techniques don't work well with stressed children because they do not provide what is needed for them to return to a state of regulation. These techniques will work better with children who have not had trauma or chronic stress in their lives. Even with "normally developed" children, though, it is important to note that one definition of *discipline* is to teach or train. I would much rather use techniques that teach and train children then punish them.

Dr. Howard Glasser's Nurtured Heart Approach: Dr. Howard Glasser, a Psychologist in Arizona, Executive Director of the Children's

Success Foundation, and author and creator of *The Nurtured Heart Approach* to difficult children, writes and speaks about children's intensity, and how we approach it. He stresses that rather than finding ways to make children's intensity go away with things like medications, the goal is to "shift the energy" instead - transforming it into success. Glasser defines success as what happens that doesn't have to, and what doesn't happen that could have. He believes that with specific intentions behind our behavior, we *can* "go in manually" and create shifts in children's behavior, even if they fit a certain profile.

Glasser's view of children is unique in that it is based on the concepts of intention, radiating energy, and creating energy shifts. These are things you typically read about in spiritual or metaphysical books. He has found a beautiful way to bring these concepts into a behavioral approach for children that works. In fact, although the research on this approach is fairly new, educational programs in Arizona that have made the Nurtured Heart Approach their foundation (such as Head Start), have witnessed *incredible* decreases in behavioral referrals and increases in successes. This is an approach well worth checking into.

Glasser teaches three basic aspects that are all about your intention, and where you put your focus, or energy, with your children:

1. super energize success experiences;
2. refuse to energize or accidentally reward negativity; and
3. provide a perfect level of limit-setting and consequences.

Essentially, Glasser explains that "what we invest our energy in is often interpreted as what we love and what we desire more of." So, the more energy you radiate around a situation, the more of a payoff the child gets from it, even if the energy exchange is negative. Typically, adults radiate much more energy around the negative than the positive. Say, for example, that your child puts their shoes where they belong without being told. You may not even acknowledge this because you *expect* it. At the most, you might say, "Good job" or "Thank you for putting your shoes away." But, if they leave their shoes in the middle of the floor, you will likely radiate a lot of energy around it, and might say very assertively, "How many times have I told you to put your shoes in your closet when you get home?... Blah,

blah, blah." There is typically much more energy around the correcting than the thanking. One key to transforming a child's behavior, according to Glasser, is to shift where you radiate the most energy.

In his book, *The Nurtured Heart Approach*, Glasser details what can be called "energizing success." In this phase, he explains four goals to transforming children's behavior:

1. Move beyond "catching them being good," and *create* space or opportunities for them to succeed.
2. Radiate as much energy as you can around their successes.
3. Radiate as little energy as you can around negativity.
4. Provide rewards and limits in the right places, at the right levels.

Move beyond "catching them being good," and *create* space or opportunities for your child to succeed. Glasser refers to this as *The Shamu Principle*: Shamu learns to jump over a rope in stages. During the first stage, the rope is placed on the bottom of the tank. As Shamu swims over it naturally and without effort (because he has no choice), he is rewarded just as grandly as if he had jumped through a basketball hoop. Gradually, and with much rewarding for success, the rope is raised up, until eventually, Shamu is jumping the rope when it is held 10 feet above the water. This is about *creating* space for your child to be successful, with little or no effort, and then, giving them a taste of how it feels to have all of your positive energy radiated at them around it. In this way, they will want to "come back for more." This sets the stage for the shift to take place from rewarding the negative to rewarding the positive.

Radiate as much energy as you can around your child's successes. Every time your child does something positive, or chooses not to do something negative, make a fuss. Let them know that they have been seen, noticed, and valued when they are not acting out. You do not have to wait until something great has happened. Narrate or describe what you see your child doing – out loud. Your comments should simply reflect what you observe without judgment or question. Pay attention to their actions and their emotions. For example, "You are really putting a lot of thought into how to solve that math problem," or "I can tell that you are really having fun with your rollerblades."

This is your way of verbally documenting each moment, as if taking a snapshot of your child. If your child gets angry or acts out more when you start this, Glasser says this means that they like the attention and are reverting back to their old way of how to keep it (by acting out). Instead of doing less noticing, this is your clue to do more. At this point, your child does not yet trust that they can hold your attention with successes.

Radiate as little energy as you can around your child's negativity. Do not make the mistake of lecturing your child after they have made a negative choice. This has the opposite effect of accidentally energizing what you do not want. Instead of making a fuss around the behavior that you do not want your child to continue, radiate the energy around the behaviors that you want your child to continue. Verbally recognize, appreciate and fuss over your child when they show you the values you are trying to teach them. For example, "I like how you are being successful. Let me tell you how I see you being successful right now…" Again, you are providing your child with snapshots of how and when they are successful.

Provide rewards and limits in the right places, at the right levels. Glasser compares this skill to the structure of a computer game: the rules and incentives are completely clear and predictable. There are clear and immediate rewards for making successful choices (for example, points), and when a rule is broken, the message is simple: "Oops. Broke a rule. There is a consequence." No fuss, no energy radiated around it; that round, or turn, is simply over. Then, you use what you've learned and can try again. The motivation to try again is born out of the stockpiling of rewards for correct moves, and the lack of shame for wrong moves.

It is important to appreciate when your child does not break the rules. For instance, "I love that you didn't… today," or "I applaud you for not…" This, in essence, is giving them "game points" for making the right moves. In this way, you are acknowledging their moments of success, while at the same time, giving a warning about what is not allowed. This also sets the stage for rules and consequences to really have an effect. Glasser suggests that rather than relying on positive language for your rules (which generally works with average children), state them in a way that leaves no doubt about what is *not* allowed (which generally works best with challenging children). For example, "No eating in your bedroom."

Three: Parent Beliefs and Expectations

We all use what others show us about ourselves as a mirror for who we are and how we are doing. That's why the beliefs and expectations you hold about your child are so powerful. Children judge themselves by what you mirror to them about who they are and what they are capable of. Parent beliefs and expectations is a third area of your parenting to review for fine-tuning.

Even well-intended parents can hold negative beliefs or expectations that are revealed to children through words and gestures. Just by having these beliefs, we give them the force they need to become reality. For example, if you believe that your child cannot learn to ride a bike, then chances are, they will not learn to ride a bike. They will absorb the "force" of your belief, even if you do not speak it, because there is no way to contain or conceal the energy that is behind that belief. It will come out somehow in your words or gestures. Many children are sensitive enough to pick up on this energy, even when we try to hide it. They will meet our expectations almost every time, whether these expectations are positive or negative.

The exception to this (and there always is one) is the child who is strong-willed enough to decide that they will do it anyway, even if no one believes that they can. Some children simply make up their minds that they will do the opposite of what others expect or believe of them. Whether this is strength, confidence, stamina, or rebellion, who knows? But wouldn't it be nice to be "on the same side" as your child, rather than in a constant power struggle with them? If you hold positive beliefs about your children and always support their efforts, they will develop the confidence to try their best at everything.

At the same time, it is important for children to learn that it is okay if they cannot do something the way they would like to. We are humans. We are not perfect. We make mistakes. We learn from our mistakes and attempts, and we use them to become smarter and stronger.

By developing a willingness to try, children can learn that mistakes, "failures", or unsuccessful attempts are important opportunities to learn and grow, rather than something to be ashamed of.

Beware of having expectations that are unreasonably high, though. This can create the feeling of hopelessness and overwhelm in children. They may feel like no matter what they do or how hard they try, it is never good enough. Children need to feel that they are loved and accepted just the way they are. This does not mean that encouragement should be avoided. Later in this section, we will look more closely at ways to encourage children that build self-esteem and independence (rather than insecurity and dependence). Also, your standards for children's behavior must match their age and developmental abilities. Otherwise, they can become discouraged.

Another trap that parents sometimes fall into is encouraging competition among brothers and sisters. Parents may praise one child's success and ignore or criticize the other child. They may overlook a valiant attempt by a child that meant as much to them as success itself might have. In this situation, children may judge themselves as incapable of succeeding at things that their sibling does well. They may do the opposite, do nothing at all, or choose something that has not been tried by their sibling instead. When parents encourage all their children in whatever they try, competition between siblings lessens, and they begin to find their place in the family without feeling a need to overshadow or compete with each other.

Sometimes parents are overambitious in wanting their children to be their best all the time. Expecting children to be excellent in every situation teaches them not to attempt things unless they think they will be successful at it, so as not to disappoint their parents. They may avoid trying certain things out of a fear of failure. They may become perfectionists or be overly self-critical or negative of their attempts. They may be afraid to admit their imperfections or mistakes, and will likely put extreme pressure on themselves. Parents may unwittingly encourage these patterns by making simple comments like, "Keep up the good work." Children can interpret this to mean that they are not good enough or that they must always be perfect to be loved.

Remember that children's behavior is most influenced by *your* behavior. If you have certain expectations of your children, they will learn these best by following your role model. For instance, if you tell your children one thing, yet you do another, they will do what you do, *not* what you say. If you do not want your child to smoke cigarettes or drink alcohol, yet you smoke and drink in their presence, chances are they will smoke and drink when they get the opportunity. This type of double standard can also give children the feeling that they do not have as much value in the family as others do. In reality, they are just as important as everybody else. If you allow yourself the privilege of rest time between work and doing household chores, for example, your child deserves the same privilege after school.

To avoid these traps, Don Dinkmeyer and Gary McKay suggest that parents:

1.   accept their children as they are, not only as they could be;
2.   ignore tattling since it is used to look good or get even;
3.   have faith in their children so they will believe in themselves;
4.   focus on children's contributions, assets, and strengths;
5.   recognize children's efforts and growth, as well as mastery;
6.   respect children; this is the foundation for developing self-respect;
7.   encourage instead of praise (See Four below);
8.   be positive; use active, reflective listening; I-messages; problem-solving; and natural and logical consequences instead of negativity (See Five, Six, Seven, and Eight below).

Four: Supporting with Encouragement instead of Praise

A fourth area of parenting that contributes to children's behavior is how they are supported. This goes along with parental attitudes and expectations. Support can be given in a way that builds self-esteem and encourages internal motivation (encouragement), or it can be given in a way that weakens self-esteem and encourages external motivation (praise). The difference between these two styles will become more clear as you read the examples below.

Basically, praise is a type of social control. Its purpose is to reward children for what parents consider "good" behavior. There is judgment attached to praise. The message is, "I will reward you with praise and attention when you do good, because you only have value when you do good." With praise, children hear, "my worth depends on how you (and others) judge me."

Encouragement, on the other hand, is meant to make a child feel valuable for their efforts, their growth, and for having the courage to try. There is no external judgment attached to it, so children learn to trust and rely on their self-evaluation. This also teaches them to rely on their own decisions. Encouragement can be given any time, not just when children are successful. The message is, "You are capable and have value no matter what happens." Children hear, "My efforts are important and I have value even when I do not succeed. My worth depends on how I judge myself."

Consider these differences between praise and encouragement:

Underlying Characteristics	What Child May Hear or Perceive	Possible Results
Praise: Focus is on external control.	"I am worthwhile only when I do what you want."	Child learns to measure worth by ability to conform; or, child rebels (views cooperation as giving in).
Encouragement: Focus is on internal control and the child's ability to manage life constructively.	"I am trusted to become responsible and independent."	Child learns courage to be imperfect and willingness to try; gains self-confidence and comes to feel responsible for own behavior.
Praise: Focus is more on external evaluation.	"To be worthwhile I must please you." "Please or perish."	Child learns to measure worth on how well (s)he pleases others, and to fear disapproval.

Underlying Characteristics	What Child May Hear or Perceive	Possible Results
Encouragement: Focus is on internal evaluation.	"How I feel about myself and my own efforts is most important."	Child learns to evaluate own progress and to make own decisions.
Praise: Is rewarded only for well-done, completed tasks.	"To be worthwhile, I must meet your standards."	Child develops unrealistic standards, learns to measure worth by how closely (s)he reaches perfection, and learns to dread failure.
Encouragement: Recognizes effort and improvement.	"I don't have to be perfect. My efforts and improvements are important."	Child learns to accept efforts of self and others, and develops desire to stay with tasks (persistence.)
Praise: Focuses on self-evaluation and personal gain.	"I'm the best. I must continue to be better than others to be worthwhile."	Child learns to be overcompetitive, to get ahead at others' expense; feels worthwhile only when "on top."
Encouragement: Focuses on assets, contributions, and appreciation.	"My contribution counts. I am appreciated."	Child learns to use talents and efforts for good of all, not only for personal gain; and to feel glad for successes of others as well as for own successes.

Adapted from Dinkmeyer & McKay (1989) STEP: The Parent's Handbook.

Remember: the keys to giving encouraging statements are:

1.   Focus on the word "You" instead of "I."

2. Be specific instead of general: "You are working hard to write neatly" instead of "Nice job."

3. Do not say things that carry judgment, like, "It's about time!" or "Why couldn't you do that before?" or "You should have..."

Lynn Lott, M.A., M.F.C.C., and Jane Nelsen, Ed.D., M.F.C.C., developed a manual for facilitating parenting support classes called, *Teaching Parenting the Positive Discipline Way.* They are certified marriage and family counselors in private practice, and have been writing, teaching, speaking, and doing workshops on parenting since 1969. Their parenting manual provides us with some specific examples of how to change praise statements into encouraging statements. Here are a few to consider:

Praise	Encouragement
I'm proud of you!	You can be proud of yourself! I appreciate your help.
You are so smart!	You figured it out!
You always know the right answer.	I have faith in you.
You did it perfectly.	You worked hard.
That's my girl/boy!	You reached your goal!
With more work, you'll get it right.	I trust your judgment.
You know what I like.	You are capable.
Good job!	You are dependable.
You're the best player on the team.	You did your best.

You got an A!	Look what you learned!
I'm impressed.	Look at your progress.
You're better than that.	You decide for yourself.
I like it.	Keep at it; You made it!
That's what I expected.	You did what you wanted.

Five: Open instead of Closed Communication

A fifth area of parenting that influences children's behavior is looking at how you communicate with them. Effective communication involves two parts: how you listen and how you speak. For example, an open style of listening means that you hear and accept the child's feelings, you understand their meanings, and that you give them your full attention by facing them and making eye contact. This gives them the message that what they are saying has importance and is worth your attention, which means that *they* are important and are worth your attention. It also tells children that you respect them and their feelings. This type of listening is called "active listening."

In contrast, a closed style of listening tells children that they are not important. This involves not making eye contact, not giving them your full attention, and not reflecting their feelings to give a sense of understanding and acceptance. This style of listening is called "passive listening" and is a sure way to shut down the channels of communication between you and your child.

How you respond to your child is just as important as how you listen to them. For instance, an open style of speaking (or responding) means that you avoid the negative, like nagging, criticizing, threatening, lecturing, probing, commanding, judging, preaching, and ridiculing. It also means that you resist the urge to give a solution, but walk them through the steps of problem solving, instead. This teaches them to take responsibility for their actions and evaluate consequences. There is one exception here: if children are discussing something that could be hurtful to themselves or to someone else. In this case, you can still walk them through problem solving, but keeping everyone safe is the ultimate goal.

What you want to do instead is reflect the child's feelings and meanings back to them so that they feel heard and understood. In counseling, this is called "reflective listening" since you are being a "mirror" for your child's feelings so that they can "see" themselves more clearly. Responding in an open style supports the development of problem-solving, confidence, and competence in children. Just as with closed listening, though, a closed style of responding tells children that you have not heard, accepted, or understood their feelings. Children will feel unimportant and they will eventually stop talking to you about personal issues.

Here are a few examples of what each looks like:

Closed Response	Open Response
Why not forget it; they probably didn't mean it.	You're really angry with them.
Now, don't talk like that! You just got started!	It seems very hard to you.
We've talked about this before so stop fussing.	It seems unfair to you.
That's nice...now will you please go so that I can...	You're pleased with your work on it. You are proud!
Everyone has to do it.	You're afraid of getting hurt.
Don't you ever talk to me that way!	You're very angry with me.

Adapted from Dinkmeyer & McKay (1989) STEP: The Parent's Handbook .

If you are not practicing open communication, it is never too late to start. The more you practice, the easier and more natural it will feel. You should begin to see some differences within a week or two, if you use open communication consistently. To sum up, when your child is talking to you, you *don't want* to judge, criticize, blame, name-call, ridicule, shame, interpret, diagnose, analyze, solve, teach, or instruct. You *want* to listen, attend, make eye contact, reflect feelings, encourage, acknowledge, and support.

Six: I-Messages Instead of You-Messages

Understanding the difference between an "I-message" and a "You-message" is a sixth area of parenting to consider. The I-message looks like this: "I feel (this way) when (this happens), and (here are the choices). This process accomplishes three goals: it tells how you feel, it tells what makes you feel that way, and it tells what can be changed to remedy the situation. This takes the guesswork out for the child. For those times when children need to be confronted about their behavior, I-messages foster safety and openness, while discouraging defensiveness. There is no blame in an I-message, so there is little defensiveness. Blame leads to shame and guilt, which leads to defensiveness. With an I-message, you are simply stating the facts about how you feel, why you feel that way, and what would help you feel better. This makes it easier for children to hear what you are saying and be more willing to try to find a solution.

In contrast to I-messages, You-messages are "you-oriented." They say, "You did this" and "You did that." The feeling that You-messages typically convey is anger, and the message that is sent to the child is blame. Blame eventually becomes shame, guilt and defensiveness.

Some examples of You-messages versus I-messages are:

You-Message	I-Message
(You) Stop playing that so loud!	I can't work with loud noise. Turn it down or listen in your room.

You-Message	I-Message
You are acting like a baby.	I am too tired to do that now.
Why don't you behave?	I'm worried about it breaking. Treat it gently or play with something else.
You know better than that!	I'm upset that it broke.
(You) Don't do that!	I'm worried about finishing on time. Push the cart or sit down.

Usually, an I-message will disarm a child. If a child lashes out after an I-message, your best bet is not to take it personally. Instead, realize that they are struggling, fearful, and defensive, and it may be best to simply give them some space and your blessings. Remember: children do as we do, not as we say. Continue to use open communication with them so that they will know you are there for them when they choose to reconnect with you. This is a good opportunity to model mature, loving behavior during tense times.

Sometimes, children ignore I-messages, especially when parents first use them. It may be hard for them to hear how their behavior makes someone else feel. When this happens, use a second I-message, and/or say something to get the child's attention: "Mary, this is important to me. I'm telling you how I feel." If your child responds to your I-message with one of their own, shift into reflective listening so they will feel understood and accepted. For example:

Child: "Well, I'm too tired to wash the dishes!"
You: "You must have had a very busy day at school today."

When you practice I-messages, remember that they focus on *how you feel*, without blaming the child. You can add some behavioral choices for them if you would like, or simply express how you feel. Many children respond positively to this shift. Be careful not to "dress a You-message in I-message clothing." For example, consider this situation borrowed from Dr. Thomas Gordon's book, *P.E.T: Parent Effectiveness Training*: "I get angry when you goof off and neglect your chores." In one sentence, the child was called a goof off and neglectful. Instead, consider this: "I worry that the garbage will not get picked up." As with the other skills reviewed in this chapter, mastery of using I-messages becomes easier with practice.

Seven: Problem Solving

A seventh way that parents can encourage more harmony in their relationship with children is through the use of problem solving. It is a form of active listening that teaches children to become more responsible for their choices and accepting of consequences. In general, problem solving involves walking your child through five steps:

1. Defining or identifying the problem;
2. Freely brainstorming solutions without judgment;
3. Discussing possible consequences attached to each solution considered in step 2;
4. Choosing one to try and deciding when to try it;
5. Reviewing the outcome and deciding if further action must be taken.

Although this process can be done with words alone, I recommend writing each step down for memory's sake. Then, the document can be revisited and revised as needed during step 5. It can also serve as a good reminder in the future of what has already been tried and whether it was helpful or not.

"Think Aloud," a popular program for teaching problem solving skills to children, was specifically designed with impulsive youngsters in mind. It is a problem-solving model aimed at teaching impulse control through speech, or "verbal mediation." Children are taught to, literally, think out loud while solving problems. They review and complete each step in the process out loud. As a result, the problem-solving steps become more automatic. Once children show mastery of the steps, they are encouraged to transfer this skill inward, into their minds – first with a whisper, then mentally to themselves, in silence. Bonnie Camp, M.D., Ph.D., Professor of Pediatrics and Psychiatry at the Colorado School of Medicine, co-developed the Think Aloud program for use with children in the schools. She describes the four problem solving steps in the program as follows:

1. *Identify the problem:* Children will need to have a clear understanding of the problem. Use the cue question, "What am I supposed to do?" or "What is bothering me?"

2. *Develop and choose a plan:* Model the way to list several possibilities, and use the cue question, "What are some plans?"

3. *Monitor performance:* Check on how well the chosen plan is being followed. Use the cue question, "Am I using my plan?" When teaching this skill to children, it is important to model mistakes, and how to correct them or revise the plan.

4. *Evaluate the outcome:* Check on how well the plan worked, and whether it was safe, fair, and kind. Use the cue question, "How did I do?" or "Did my plan work?"

Betty Youngs, an expert in the field of managing stress, suggests this four-step plan that is similar to the "Think Aloud" model:

1. *"What's my problem?"* Help the child specifically define the issue.

2. *"How can I solve it?"* Help the child brainstorm all possible solutions.

3. *"What's my plan?"* Let the child select what they think is the best solution, and then talk about how to put the plan into action.

4. *"How did I do?"* Help the child review how it went, and what they might do differently next time.

These programs are intended to be easy to remember, and to strengthen youngsters' ability to think before they act. The focus is on getting students to recall and use the four "self-instruction," or cue, questions on their own. These methods have been used successfully with students in elementary, secondary, and high school. Remember the old saying that goes something like, "If the hungry come to you for fish, do not *give* them fish; give them a pole and *teach* them to fish." The same principle applies here: rather than trying to solve your child's problems for them, consider modeling and teaching them how to do it successfully for themselves. Both of you will be thankful that you did.

Eight: The Goals of Behavior

The eighth area of parenting to consider is learning about the goals of children's behavior. It is important to remember that *all* behavior is goal-driven rather than random; human behavior always has a social purpose. In the mid 20th century, Dr. Rudolf Dreikurs, an American psychiatrist, proposed that people misbehave when one of four basic human needs are not met: attention, power, revenge, and avoidance of failure. Later, psychologists Don Dinkmeyer and Gary McKay linked this principle to faulty beliefs about the self:

Goal of Misbehavior	Faulty Belief
Attention (to keep others busy or to get special attention)	I belong only when I am being noticed or getting special service. I am only important when I am keeping you busy with me.
Power (to be boss)	I belong only when I am in control or am boss, or when I am proving that no one can boss me.
Revenge (to get even)	I belong only by hurting others as I feel hurt. I cannot be liked or loved.
Assumed Inadequacy or Avoidance of Failure (to give up and be left alone)	I do not believe I can belong, so I will convince others not to expect anything from me. I am helpless and unable. It is no use trying because I will not do it right.

Adapted from Dinkmeyer & McKay (1989) STEP: The Parent's Handbook.

Knowing these goals and beliefs is an important key to unweaving your child's misbehavior. Once you are aware of their goals and the faulty beliefs supporting them, you can take steps to shift them. In most situations, your reaction to your child's behavior will reveal its true purpose:

Goal of Misbehavior	Your Feelings and Reaction
Undue Attention	Annoyed; irritated; worried; guilty; tendency to remind and coax; doing things for the child that they could do themselves
Power	Anger; challenged; threatened; defeated; fight or give in; wanting to be right; thinking, "You can't get away with it" or "I'll make you"
Revenge	Deeply hurt; disappointed; disbelieving; disgusted; tendency to retaliate or get even; taking their behavior personally; thinking, "How could you do this to me?"
Assumed inadequacy or Avoidance of Failure	Despair; hopeless; helpless; inadequate; giving up; doing for; over-helping; showing a lack of faith; agreeing with the child that nothing can be done

Adapted from Dinkmeyer & McKay (1989) STEP: The Parent's Handbook.

Children's behavior is influenced the most by *your* behavior. By shifting your responses to your child, over time you can correct their faulty beliefs about themselves and create a different pattern between the two of you:

Child's Faulty Belief	Your New response	Child's New Belief & Behavior
Undue attention: I belong only when noticed or served	Let the child know their contributions count and that you appreciate their help. Involve them in useful and fun tasks.	I belong by contributing Helps; volunteers
Power: I belong only when in control and the boss	Let the child experience both positive & negative outcomes; encourage their decision making; express confidence in them; offer limited choices	I can decide and be responsible for my behavior Shows self-discipline; does own work; is resourceful
Revenge: I belong only by hurting others; I cannot be loved	Let the child know you appreciate their interest in cooperating; deal with the hurt feelings; show you care; encourage their strengths; don't take behavior personally; avoid retaliation and punishment; listen with your heart	I am interested in cooperating Returns kindness for hurt; ignores belittling comments; works for fairness
Assumed inadequacy/ Avoidance of Failure: I belong only by convincing others not to expect anything from me; I am unable and helpless	Recognize their attempts to act maturely; take small steps; show faith in their abilities; don't pity; encourage all attempts; don't give up; make time to teach	I can decide to withdraw from conflict • Ignores provocations; withdraws from power contest to decide own behavior; accepts others' opinions

Adapted from Dinkmeyer & McKay (1989) STEP: The Parent's Handbook.

Taking some time to learn what is motivating your child can provide insights into what you can do to help shift their behavior. As you change your responses to them, their behavior will begin to change. This is not a "quick fix," however; it will take time, practice, and patience, as will the other skills presented in this chapter. In the long run, you will be very glad that you made an effort to understand the behavior patterns between you and your child. Unweaving these patterns and making changes in how you interact with your child will support them in feeling good about themselves, while teaching them how to get their needs met in successful and acceptable ways. Awareness is the first step toward change. Once you become aware of your child's behavior patterns and the reasons for them, you can begin to make changes that will make a long-term difference in your lives.

Nine: Getting Things Done

The Ninth area of parenting to fine-tune is your approach to getting things done in a way that is easier on both you and your child. Many children have a hard time focusing, recalling directions, following through, and completing tasks. There are many choices available to parents for managing children's behavior when things must get done. First, this is a good time to practice the communication skills we reviewed in numbers Four through Seven. Second, here are eight more ways to support your child in getting things done:

1. Make eye contact when giving a directive. Children will be more likely to follow through with a directive when you make certain they are listening to you when you give it. Turn off distractions like the television, radio, and computer. Stand before the child, instead of speaking or yelling across a room. Look them in the eyes and speak slowly and clearly. Make sure they are looking back at you. Have them repeat what they heard you say so you can make sure they got it all. Be clear and matter-of-fact.

2. Break tasks down into small steps. This makes it easier for children to remember what they are supposed to do. When they finish the first step, give them more, but never more than two at a time. Leave out extra information that may confuse or distract the child. Be calm, clear and specific. Try to plan ahead so that you will not feel pressured to rush them.

No: (Parent yells from nearby.) "Jane, turn off the T.V., it's time to go! Put your socks on, and wear your tennis shoes because we will be outside. Bring them to me and I will help you tie them. Then, we can leave. Hurry! We don't have much time!"

YES: (Parent turns T.V. off and makes eye contact.) "Jane, we have ten minutes to get to the party. It's time for you to find your socks and put them on." (When Jane returns), "Now, bring me your tennis shoes." (Helps Jane put on shoes.) "Now, it's time to go!"

Of course, this is a simplified example, but you get the idea. Avoid arguing with your child if they whine or complain. Instead, rely on some of the communication skills we reviewed earlier, such as reflective listening. Remember, practice makes perfect.

3. Take time to teach and give time to learn. If you ask your child to do something new at home, be sure you take the time to walk them through it at least once before allowing them to do it on their own. Modeling your expectations of how to accomplish a task makes it easier for children to remember. This will also prevent any arguments or disagreements over how it is to be done. Avoid urges to help or correct them. Instead, allow them to make choices and decisions on their own, and learn from the results. Make sure you give them plenty of time to learn and complete the task. Rushing children can distract and frustrate them. Consider ways to allow them to complete things at their own pace.

Keep in mind that we only retain 20% of what we hear, but we remember 30% of what we see, 50% of what we hear *and* see, 70% of what we say, and 90% of what we say *and* do. Here is another great opportunity to practice some of the skills reviewed earlier: Model aloud your process for making decisions about how to do something so they can learn from your demonstration, including mistakes! Have them repeat the steps back to you. Encourage and support your child's attempts at doing new or different things. Use your reflective and active listening skills if they become frustrated or unsure of themselves. Letting children know that you trust them and are confident in their abilities can boost their self-esteem and help them feel more secure in trying new things.

4. Give choices or tasks that match the child's level of development. Be sure that what you are asking the child to do is something that they understand and are capable of doing or learning to do. If they are given a task that is beyond their capabilities, they may become angry, frustrated, upset, or rebellious. They may feel incompetent and negative or critical toward themselves. They may choose not to try anything else that they are uncertain of. That is why it is very important to make certain that what you are asking the child to do is within their learning zone. Start with a few simple tasks that you *know* your child can do on their own, and give lots of encouragement. This builds confidence. Avoid criticizing or correcting their "work." They will be more willing to help if they know that you respect their decisions and abilities. If they *ask* you what you think, use reflective listening or ask them what *they* think:

NO: "Well, this part is crooked. And you didn't…(blah, blah, blah). I can't trust you with anything. You never do it right!"

YES: "You're wondering if you did it right. How comfortable are *you* with it?" or "What would you change?" or "What do you see that may be different than what I showed you?" or "Which part are you not sure about?" and "You worked hard at it."

You can make checking their work part of the teaching process while they are learning. Then, it will be easier for you to talk with them about their progress. If they need more coaching and practice, use open-ended questions and encourage *them* to identify the problem areas. Remember that they are learning. Their skills will improve over time, and once mastery is established, no checking will be . needed. Encourage *all* attempts!

5. Keep visual reminders around the house. Remember, we only retain 20% of what we hear and 30% of what we see, but we retain 50% of what we see and hear. This is why it is so helpful to both tell and show children what to do. Posting visual cues, or reminders, in a special spot (or spots) in the house will make it easier for your child to complete what they are asked to. And, you will not have to serve as their memory. For example, simply list the things they are responsible for on a sheet of paper with easy-to-follow instructions. Feel free to include pictures, get creative, use color, and have fun with this. Just be sure that it is clear, specific, and in an obvious spot in the house. If they help you create it, it will hold more meaning for them, and they will be more likely to remember the list.

6. Allow for short breaks. For children with a lot of energy, it is often helpful to allow them to take a short break from their task every 15-30 minutes or so. The break can be as short as five minutes and no more than 10 minutes, or they may have difficulty returning to the task. Discuss with them beforehand what they might like to do during their breaks, and agree on a few choices. Trials may be necessary to fine-tune these. Using a timer is a big help for monitoring the breaks. Although this works very well with some children, no one knows your child as well as you do. Use your judgment and be willing to experiment.

7. Keep distractions to a minimum. Try to remove things that will distract your child from what they are supposed to be doing. Turn off the television; turn down the music; ask other children to go into another room; put away toys; etc. Chances are that if they see a more attractive choice, they will go for it! The goal is to provide enough calm and structure for them to focus on the task long enough to get it done.

8. Make logical consequences as immediate as possible. Be sure your child knows what the household rules are, and what the consequences are for breaking them. If they have a specific job to do at home and they fail to do it, enforce the logical consequence as soon as you know. This should be something that has been decided ahead of time and discussed with your child at a neutral time, so that there is no question about whether or not they knew and understood the process. Remember to be consistent.

Some Final Thoughts

There are many, many parenting resources out there in books, videos, magazines, etc. In this chapter, I have summarized the main points from some of my favorites. You are the expert on your child, however, and are in the best position to know what strategies are likely to help and which ones probably will not help. It is impossible for anyone to know what will work for *all* children or *all* parents, because they are each unique and living in unique situations. But we can develop parenting tools that support healthy growth and personal responsibility for children. My hope is that you found something useful in this chapter to bring a bit more ease, relaxation, and harmony into your relationship with your child.

4

"IF THIS, THEN THAT"

Teaching children to make responsible choices

THE ABILITY TO think through actions before taking them is a skill that can help children make choices to support their success in life. As parents, we want our children to understand that each of their choices has results. We want them to move through the world with self-awareness, and to learn to take responsibility for their actions. This skill comes more naturally for some than for others. The good news is that it can be learned. In this chapter, I share different ways parents can support children in making more thoughtful, responsible choices. This information is especially helpful for children who show more severe or challenging behaviors, or who have a difficult time managing even basic interactions in a successful way.

Teaching with Natural and Logical Consequences

Teaching style (or discipline) is the area of parenting typically used to shift children's behavior. Many parenting books stress the use of natural and logical consequences when teaching or disciplining children, instead of rewards and punishment. There are many reasons for this, although I believe an important one is that natural and logical consequences teach children to be responsible for their own choices and the consequences of those choices. This is an important life skill that kids can use forever. In contrast, the reward and punishment model of discipline requires parents to be responsible for kids' choices. Other major differences between these two discipline styles are listed below:

Reward & Punishment	Natural & Logical Consequences
Parents are responsible for the child's behavior	Children are responsible for their own behavior
Children are prevented from learning to make their own decisions	Children learn to make their own decisions
Acceptable behavior is only needed when adults are present as enforcers	Children learn acceptable behavior from the consequences of their own choices, whether adults are present or not
Invites resistance and rebellion by forcing conformity	Children can only evaluate themselves and their choices
Emphasizes the power of personal authority	Emphasizes natural social order, mutual rights, and mutual respect
Tends to be arbitrary or unrelated to the situation	Directly related to the situation
Personal and involves judgment	Impersonal and without judgment
Concerned with past behavior	Concerned with present and future behavior
Threatens disrespect or loss of love	Neutral and matter-of-fact
Demands obedience	Permits choice

Adapted from Dinkmeyer & McKay (1989) STEP: The Parent's Handbook.

Natural consequences allow children to learn from the natural order of things, or the reality of nature. For instance, if your child leaves their bike outside over night and it rusts in the rain or is stolen, this is a natural consequence. Rather than reminding and coaxing your child to put the bike away, allow the natural order of things to "do the dirty work." Natural consequences tend to work no matter what the child's behavioral goal is.

Logical consequences allow children to learn from the social order of things, or the reality of the social world. For example, if you have a rule that bikes must be put away over night, and your child leaves their bike out over night, you can remove the privilege of using the bike for a reasonable and meaningful period of time (assuming that the child knew the rule and the consequence for breaking it beforehand). This puts the responsibility and choice on the child, since they knew what the rule was, and what the consequence was for breaking the rule. The consequence for not putting the bike away flows logically from the child's choice. Logical consequences are more effective for attention-getting behavior, and less effective when the child's goal is power or revenge.

Remember, when applying consequences:

1. **Provide choices:** "You can turn that down or turn it off. You decide which you would rather do."

2. **Leave room for change:** "I see you have chosen to turn that off by not lowering the volume. Feel free to turn it back on when you are ready to lower the volume."

3. **If the child repeats the misbehavior, be prepared to extend the amount of time required between tries (this means they are not ready to be responsible):** "I see that you are still not ready to turn that down and have decided to turn it off. You can try again tomorrow afternoon."

4. **Be consistent and follow-through with rules and decisions:** "I see that after trying again today, you are still not ready to lower the volume and have decided to turn it off. You can try again the day after tomorrow."

Keep in mind that discipline is one way to show your child that you care. The goal is not to hurt, humiliate, or manipulate children, but rather, to teach them to be responsible for their choices and behavior. Discipline methods that do not work can result in hurt feelings, confusion, lowered self-esteem, manipulative behavior, fear, insecurity, and difficulty coping. Instead, focus your attention on methods that teach, empower, and support your child in becoming a healthy, responsible person.

Things That Show You Care and Work	Things That Hurt and Do Not Work
Anticipating and planning	Spanking
Being clear and consistent	Yelling
Practicing	Sarcasm
Setting limits	Labeling
Giving and respecting choices	Making threats or promises
Following through with natural and logical consequences	Using unrealistic consequences
	Rejecting
Being calm, firm, and matter-of-fact	Isolating
Presenting a united front (if there are two of you),	Ignoring
	Terrorizing
Being a role model	Manipulating
Dealing with one child at a time	Degrading

When delivering consequences, consider these final suggestions:

1. Use a friendly, matter-of-fact tone of voice; be firm and kind.

2. Show an open, accepting attitude; set limits, provide choices, allow the child to decide how to respond to them, and accept their decision. Your goal is not to win or control, but to teach them responsibility for their behavior.

3. Be sure the consequence is logically related to the misbehavior.

4. Separate the misbehavior from the child: "I love you, and I am upset about this mess!"

5. Say as little as possible and focus on following through with consequences.

6. Pick your battles carefully; let minor behaviors slide until major behaviors shift; use positive comments.

Psychology's "Contingency Theory" for Shifting Behavior

There is an area of psychology that focuses on understanding what drives human behavior. Part of what this area researches is known as "contingency theory." Contingency theory basically says that human behavior is often driven by the knowledge that "if this happens, then that will follow." This theory is a twist on the old "reward and punishment" model of discipline. Researchers found that using contingencies with children can help them understand that what they choose to do in the moment determines what happens next. Contingencies are especially useful for dealing with challenging behaviors that happen often and are moderate to severe in nature.

The theory is that by using contingencies, children can learn to choose behaviors that help them succeed and avoid behaviors that don't. Contingencies are considered a form of discipline set up to:

1. support children's behavior that you want to increase;

2. acknowledge steps toward behavior that you want children to learn;

3. ignore minor misbehavior that you want to decrease; and

4. give a consequence for moderate to serious misbehavior.

Two basic concepts in psychology that reflect this model of discipline and teaching are known as "positive reinforcement" and "response cost." To support behavior you want your child to show more of, you can practice positive reinforcement. In its simplest form, positive reinforcement means noticing your child each time they do a behavior you want them to keep doing. The message the child gets is, "When you do this, you get something you like." This can take the form of praise, clapping, smiling, giving a toy or treat, or doing anything that feels good to your child. Any combination of physical things that they can hold, collect or see (like points, stickers, treats, toys, money) and things that they cannot necessarily hold, collect or see (like social or activity-based things, attention, free time, privileges, special time with a parent, special outings, hugs, pats, or verbal statements) can be used.

To discourage behavior you want your child to stop doing, you can practice response cost. Response cost means that your child loses a certain amount of a privilege they already have, every time they do something that they are not allowed to do. For example, your child may start each day with the privilege of watching 60 minutes of TV in the evening after supper. Minutes can either be added or subtracted throughout the day, depending on their behavior.

You can use a range of mild to more extreme costs, depending on the intensity and severity or danger level of the behavior. Mild costs might include ignoring, attending to a sibling who is making positive choices, leaving the room, or removing a privilege. More extreme costs could include a Time Away (explained in the next section) or restitution (assigning them a task that makes amends).

In contingency theory, there are certain concepts that can help you decide what to do for increasing, maintaining, or decreasing a behavior. Here are some examples:

CONCEPT	PURPOSE
Continuous Reinforcement	Acknowledge your child every time (s)he shows a behavior you want to see more of; this is best for strengthening new or developing behaviors.
Intermittent Reinforcement	Acknowledge a behavior some, but not every, time it is shown; this is best for behaviors that your child is already doing fairly regularly that you want them to keep doing.
Behavioral Shaping	Acknowledge every attempt and step your child makes at trying to learn a new behavior; by noticing each step in the "right" direction, the behavior is "shaped" so that your child will begin to learn the steps toward the goal, and will want to do it more.
Extinction	Pay no attention to behaviors that you want your child to stop doing; when extinction is used correctly, the behavior should gradually decrease in how often and how intensely they show it, after a temporary increase; as your child tries to pull you back into old habits, behavior may increase or intensify for a week or two before decreasing.

In the rest of this chapter, you will learn some contingency-based tools that psychology calls "behavioral management strategies." I have chosen a few strategies to share that are well researched. These include: Time Out versus Time Away, redirection, contingency contracts, self-management strategies, and token economy systems. These are techniques you can begin to practice right now, if you choose to. Remember that contingency- based tools are best suited for behaviors that are moderate to severe in level of intensity and danger.

Time Out Versus Time Away

A commonly used strategy for children's misbehavior is known as the Time Out technique. The goal of this technique is to remove the child from the situation where the misbehavior occurred until they can return to it calmly and ready to "play nice." From the Time Out technique was born "Time Away," which is a kinder, gentler version of Time Out. In a Time Away, the misbehaving child is given the space to take "Time Away" from a situation until they decide that they are ready to return. It's a more self-directed and problem-solving technique than Time Out tends to be. Let's look at each method more closely.

"Time Out" strategies have been around for years. They originated in the field of psychology and became a way to support cooperation in children. Unfortunately, they are often misused, ineffective, and punishing. For this reason, I encourage parents to use them only in desperate situations, and then, only when:

1.   the process is applied to one or two recurring, specific and severe situations;

2.   the process is explained to the child;

3.   the process is modeled for the child and rehearsed with the child long before it is tried; and

4.   parents can identify an appropriate place in the house to enforce it.

To use the Time Out strategy effectively, follow these guidelines:

1. Time Out is generally used when, even after a warning, non-compliance and/or severe misbehavior continues.

2. Time Out is generally more effective in a "contained room" where a chair can be used. Do not use the child's bedroom. Do not do it in a room with toys or other fun distractions.

3. Ideally, the chair is in a corner, facing a wall, but far enough away from the wall and other objects that they cannot be kicked or touched by the child. A straight-backed, dinette-style chair works best.

4. Ideally, the chair is within eye-shot of the parent, who stays busy in a nearby room. There is no interaction with the child during the Time Out, not even eye contact, except for safety.

5. The rule of thumb for how long a Time Out should last is one to two minutes for each year of the child's age, depending on the severity of the behavior, but no longer than 15 minutes. Some models suggest that a child stay in Time Out until they are physically and verbally calm for at least 30 seconds, regardless of age.

6. Many people find that the use of a timer calms children down in this situation. Some people suggest giving the child control over setting and turning off the timer. Other people suggest that the timer only be started after the child is physically and verbally calm.

7. If a child refuses to go to the Time Out chair, or to stay in the chair once there, some methods suggest that they be physically guided or placed there. Parents can stand behind the chair, squat down, and wrap their arms around the back of the chair, and the child's arms and waist, to hold them there. From this position, parents cannot be kicked or hit with the child's feet or head. This is called "holding." Parents can let go when the child gets calm.

8. There are two models for releasing a child from Time Out. The first suggests that parents be responsible for the release. When the child completes their time and is calm for at least 30 seconds, they should agree to follow through with any requests

made by parents before the Time Out. Otherwise, they cannot get up. The second model suggests that children monitor their own behavior and decide when they are ready for release. This method is generally ineffective, but there are always exceptions. Some children can handle this responsibility and others cannot. Use your judgment depending on your own child's level of understanding and maturity.

Time Out can be a very effective strategy when it is done according to the guidelines presented here. It can feel somewhat punishing to a child, and sometimes parents end up feeling as if they are in a power struggle with them. Although my preference is to focus on the other preventive strategies reviewed in this chapter instead of Time Out, I recognize that sometimes more "intense" methods are needed for persistent, severe misbehavior.

The Time Out process can be separated into two levels: *non-exclusionary Time Out*, in which reinforcers are removed from the child; and *exclusionary Time Out*, in which the child is removed from the "time-in" situation. There are two types of non-exclusionary Time Outs. These include:

1. *planned ignoring* (removal of social reinforcers such as attention, verbal and physical contact, for one minute or less) and

2. *removal of reinforcement* (removal of materials the child is using for one to three minutes).

Exclusionary Time Outs are considered more intrusive to the child and are generally saved for more severe behaviors. There are three types of Exclusionary Time Outs, including:

1. *contingent observation* (in which the child is removed from the time-in situation for one minute or less, but is allowed to watch it);

2. *exclusion Time Out* (in which the child is removed from the time-in situation for up to two minutes, and is not allowed to watch it); and

3. *isolation Time Out* (in which the child is placed in a different room for up to five minutes). Time Out will not work if the

child uses it to avoid something they find unpleasant in some way.

"Time Away" is modeled after the Time Out process yet is meant for a slightly different purpose. It is not a strategy for getting kids to comply, as Time Out is. Time Away is meant to be exactly that: time away from a situation to allow a child who is misbehaving to calm down, collect their thoughts, and prepare to return and try again, if they choose to. It also gives parents time to calm down and collect their thoughts.

In brief, here is how a Time Away works:

1.   Time Away generally follows a warning and severe misbehavior. It is meant as a tool for children to learn to monitor and self-manage their own behavior. Ideally, the child will take a Time Away whenever (s)he feels the need to.

2.   Time Away can be done in any location that is separate from the focus situation. It may be helpful to review this process with the child long before it is used, and allow them to choose their special Time Away place. Parents, of course, have the final say.

3.   Time Away is not meant to punish; instead, it is meant to provide a distraction from the focus event, and time for everyone to calm down and problem solve. Parents can put themselves in Time Away when they need to, also. This gives the child a good model of when to use the skill and what it looks like.

4.   The child stays in the Time Away until (s)he is calm and decides to return and try again or do something else. For some children, this works better if a specific time is given and/or the parent lets the child know when they can return. If you use a specific time, follow the one or two minute rule for each year of a child's age, depending on the severity of the misbehavior. A timer can be used to mark the time if you want. Parents can choose to review the child's problem solving process with them before they can return.

5.   If a child refuses to go to Time Away, then they are choosing to change their behavior in that moment. If they continue or

repeat the misbehavior, parents can insist that they take a Time Away to collect themselves.

6. When the child completes their Time Away and is calm, they are free to return to the activity of their choosing, as long as parents agree. Or, parents can choose to use logical consequences here, and decide that the child must find something else to do. The severity of the misbehavior will help you choose. Keep in mind, though, that giving children a chance to change their behavior is a wonderful way to support their growth. For example, *"You can come play the game with us, or you can draw. By choosing to play the game, you have decided to play fair."*

In my opinion, the Time Away process is more aligned with the authoritative parenting style reviewed earlier (in which children are given choices and encouraged to be responsible for their own behavior), while the Time Out process fits more into the authoritarian parenting style (in which children are expected to blindly comply with parents and parents are responsible for the children's behavior). Many of the parenting strategies described in this chapter can be applied as part of the Time Away process, such as problem solving, open communication, giving choices, etc. It can be an effective way to begin teaching children how to manage their own behavior.

Redirection

The strategy called "redirection" is an expansion of the old parenting technique known simply as "distraction." It simply means distracting the child away from an activity or behavior you want them to stop and on to an acceptable one. For example, a child who wants to play with mommy's glass vase might be handed several plastic containers instead, as the vase is being removed. Redirection works like this:

1. The child does something they are not supposed to do;
2. The parent tells them to stop and gives them an alternative;
3. If the child does not shift their behavior after the parent repeats the direction, they are given a consequence.

Using the same example, then, you might give a direction to your child to put the vase down (or, you might take away the vase) and say, for example, "This is not a toy. You can play with these, instead." Then, hand your child the plastic containers to redirect their attention. You want to avoid lengthy explanations of why, because that can open the door for a power struggle. If your child fusses, try reflective responding, but avoid giving too much attention to that behavior.

If your child does not shift their behavior after being told once (or twice, at most), you would need to give a fair consequence. In this way, your directions will have more meaning to your child, and will help teach them that there are consequences to their choices. This technique is helpful for parents who feel they have lost control of their child, and are seeking a way to get some power and authority back. It is a tool for encouraging cooperation that works especially well with preschoolers. Remember that whatever you give your attention to is what your child will recreate. When more of your attention is given to your child while doing what is asked, that is what they will recreate.

Contingency Contracts

Contingency, or behavioral, contracts are just that: a contract between two or more people that says what reward(s) will be earned for doing certain things. In other words, whether or not your child gets something they want is *contingent* upon their behavior. All that a contract needs is a description of the focus behavior and a description of the reward. The contract should say who will do the behavior, what the behavior is, when the behavior is to be done, and how, exactly, it is to be done to earn the reward. The reward part of the contract tells who will monitor and control delivery of the reward, what the reward is, when the reward can be received, and how much reward can be earned.

Typically, a contract involves "delayed gratification," or the idea that when the behavior is performed on Monday, for example, it will not be rewarded until the weekend. Support can be given in the meantime by marking the contract with a check, star, sticker, or other symbol each day the focus behavior is done successfully. This is not only a way to track the week's progress, but serves as a token until the full reward is given to the child later. Here is a simple example of a contingency contract:

CONTRACT

(Jane) will:
1. set the dinner table by 5:30 p.m. Monday through Friday;
2. pick up her clean clothes from laundry room and put them away where they belong by 6 p.m. on Friday.
3. come down for supper in 5 minutes or less after one call from Mom each night.

(Mom) will:
1. mark the contract each night
2. give the reward on Saturday

REWARD:

To earn the reward, (Jane) must do all three things on time each day. After a perfect week, Mom will take Jane to the park for one hour on Saturday.

Signature: _____ Date:_____

Signature: _____ Date:_____

RECORD

M	T	W	Th	F	M	T	W	Th	F
✓	✓	✓			✓	✓	✓	✓	✓
					G	R	E	A	T!

Contracts work best when the focus behaviors are things that the child is able to do already, that are easy to watch, and that produce something you can see (e.g., finished homework, clean bedroom, folded clothes). Also, there are three guidelines to keep in mind when creating a contract:

1. First, the contract must be *fair*. The expected behavior must be in balance with the selected reward. In other words, do not over- or under-compensate the child for their efforts.

2. Second, the contract must be *clear*. There should be no confusion about what is expected by either person. All people involved in the contract should agree to it, and their signature confirms this.

3. And third, the contract must be *honest*. Both people must stick to their agreement. The reward is given how and when stated on the contract when the task or behavior is completed as noted. The reward is *not* given when the task or behavior is not completed as agreed to on the contract.

You will know when it is time to end the contract. Once your child has learned the behavior and mastered using it, they will start to feel successful, proud, capable, etc. When this happens, chances are the contract can be stopped or changed so that different behaviors can be addressed. In some cases, the child will tell the parents that they no longer need the contract. In this situation, parents make the decision either to drop the contract while continuing to watch and encourage the focus behavior, or to change the contract. It's nice to have a celebration of some kind to honor the progress a child has made to complete a contract. Another way to end a contract is to slowly shift the responsibility for monitoring it to the child. The next section talks more about this type of self-monitoring.

Self-Management Strategies

Self-management, or the ability to monitor and manage your own behavior, is an important life skill to teach children. It means that they understand how their behavior affects the people and things around them, and that they respect this connection. It means that they respect themselves, too. Mastery of self-management means that they can self-evaluate, are comfortable identifying the things about themselves that they would like to change, and are able to make those changes a reality. When children are able to manage their own behavior, rather than relying on adults to control them, they achieve a level of responsibility that allows them to be a part of society in more positive and full ways. As discussed earlier in the chapter on parenting strategies, encouraging this type of responsibility also creates more self-confidence and social competence in children, and better prepares them to make decisions and solve problems in life. A sampling of self-management strategies is outlined below.

Self-monitoring involves self-observation, self-recording, and self-assessment of behavior. There are many ways to do this. You can have an end-of-the-day review, recording, and assessment time, or you can observe and record throughout the day, with an overall review and assessment at night. Or, observations, recordings, and assessments can be done during each school period. The structure of the self-monitoring process really depends on the person completing it. Recording behaviors can be as simple as marking a "+" or a "/" in a box on a piece of paper to show whether the focus behavior occurred or not during a specified period of time. Helping your child create their own, unique way to complete this can add to the effectiveness of their program. In especially tough cases, a reward can be earned when they meet their goal.

Research shows that self-monitoring generally works. It can be used at school to increase attention in the classroom, decrease aggression and talking out, and improve academic performance. Or it can be used at home to get chores done, finish homework, or stick to routines. Children are capable of learning how to monitor their own behavior. In doing so, they become more aware of it and how it affects the world around them. This awareness makes it easier for them to shift in ways that can help them become more successful socially and academically.

Self-contracts can be used for self-management. A self-contract is created by the self, for the self, and is monitored by the self. You select the task or behavior you wish to complete, how you wish to complete it, the reward you will earn for completing it, and how the reward will be given. When the time comes, you self-deliver the reward. The reward should be something special to you that was chosen beforehand. This type of contract helps you get structured and organized when trying to do something that is challenging. You hold yourself accountable on all levels, which encourages responsibility for the self.

Parents can guide children through the steps to make their own contract. This would be a good time to practice using open communication, active and reflective listening, and problem-solving (as reviewed earlier) while helping children create and carry out their contract. It is important to make certain that the behavior the child chooses to focus on is something well within their reach so that they can have some success with it and not get discouraged. The reward provides the motivation for getting the job done. Motivation and self-discipline (and maybe a little encouragement from mom or dad) are required for this one!

Self-rewarding and consequating involve selecting a focus behavior to either increase or decrease, and them setting up a self-imposed system of reward (to increase it) or consequence (to decrease it). For example, a youth who wants to lose weight might allow ice cream as a treat on Fridays for not having any the rest of the week. Or, a youngster might decide to pay their music teacher 50¢ for each night they forget to practice their instrument. Or, if a child wants to stop pulling out their hair when they are nervous, they might wear a rubber band on their wrist and pop it once each time they notice themselves pulling on their hair. This is a simpler version of the self-contract described above.

Verbal mediation is a self-management strategy that involves talking to yourself to remind, encourage, congratulate, calm, etc. Children can learn to use "positive self-talk" when they are stressed, uncertain, or otherwise needing support. For example, when afraid to try something new, a child might repeat to him/herself, "Calm down. You can do this! Keep trying." Or, a child might tell themselves to "Be quiet" in class to avoid trouble. This process goes well with the problem solving strategies we reviewed earlier. This strategy can teach children to talk themselves through difficult situations, just like the little red engine in the storybook that said, "I think I can! I think I can! I think I can!" all the way up the hill.

Alternative responses is a form of self-management that involves doing something in place of a behavior that needs to be decreased. For example, a child who wants to stop biting their nails can squeeze their hands into a fist, put their hands in their pockets, or sit on their hands each time they catch themselves beginning to nail bite. This really is as simple as it sounds!

Massed practice is the last self-management technique that I will review. It is most effective for compulsive, habitual behaviors. It means doing an undesired behavior over and over, so that the compulsion to do it decreases. This is the old "over-practice" or "over-kill" technique. In some cases, this can be very effective; in others, not so effective. This strategy is well suited for getting rid of what can be considered compulsive behaviors. Use it selectively and with awareness, with the intent to stop compulsive or repetitive behaviors.

Token Economy Systems

For children who need motivation and/or for behaviors that are difficult to shift, parents can try a "*token economy system*." Simply put, token economy systems involve three parts: (1) the focus behavior(s) to change, (2) something to use for money (a "token"), and (3) backup rewards. If you want to use a token economy system with more than one child, these three parts must be individualized for each child or the system will not work. Let's look at the specifics of each of these.

First, the focus behaviors chosen for this system should be easy to see and measure, specific, small in number, mixed in level of difficulty, and within the child's ability level.

Second, tokens are things that are safe, tangible, durable, easy to carry and store, affordable, and readily available to the "token economist" (the adult overseeing the system). They should be things that can be given to the child right after they show the behavior you want them to show. They should be things that can be easily exchanged for backup rewards later. They should not be things that might hold value in themselves, like baseball cards, or things that can be faked, like a red tally mark. They must be things that can be kept in the control of the token economist. Some ideas include special marks, stickers, stamps, washers, checkers, poker chips, coupons, initials with a special pen, holes punched in a special card, buttons, or ribbons.

Third, backup rewards are things that can be "purchased" with the tokens, such as toys, treats, free time, coupons worth different things, special jobs, privileges, favorite snacks, allowance, or a later bedtime on weekends. Ideally, the main rewards should be items, events, or activities that are new to the child, rather then things that were available to the child before the token economy began. They *can* be naturally occurring things, like *extra* time to play a favorite game or talk on the telephone.

There are certain ethical guidelines for choosing rewards. Specifically, everyone should have free access to basic things, including meals, communication (e.g., the telephone), general comforts (e.g., clean clothing), and general privileges (e.g., social interaction). These things should *not* be used as rewards.

To use a token economy system, start by keeping the number of tokens needed to buy a backup reward *small*. This allows the child to have immediate success (gets a reward), which motivates them and helps to establish the system. This can be adjusted from then on to keep the child responding in a positive way. Make certain that the exchange rate of tokens for backup rewards stays balanced. For example, with too few tokens, the child might get discouraged because they cannot buy anything. With too many, they can stockpile them to the point of not having to do anything to buy something. Balance can be created by increasing the value of tokens and decreasing the cost of items, or increasing the prices of items and decreasing the value of tokens.

Another issue to consider is that as the child earns more tokens, they will tend to spend less on "urgent" needs (like TV time) and more on "luxury" items (like movie trips). You will want to be prepared to expand the list of luxury items as the demand for them goes up. A final consideration is this: if you raise the number of tokens needed to buy items, make sure that urgent needs cost more than luxury items. This is because if luxury items cost more, the child may not be willing to "perform" enough to buy them (and they will not show the focus behavior as much). If you are working with a group of children, one way to keep the balance between tokens and backup rewards is to auction off the backup items. Each person can bid on the items, but no one can bid more than the amount of tokens they have.

When using a token economy system, you will need to consider:

1. how the tokens will be stored and given out;

2. how tokens will be exchanged for backup rewards (e.g., create a price menu for each item);

3. how to motivate the unmotivated child (e.g., allow the natural consequence of not earning enough tokens to buy anything to take effect, and encourage them to try again);

4. how to handle the child that tests the system (e.g., involve them in the planning and use; tell them that it is their choice; review the backup rewards with their input);

5. whether you will remove tokens for inappropriate behavior ("response cost"); and

6. how you plan to end the system.

Before starting a token economy system, be sure to verbally review how the system will work with the child, model how the tokens will be given, and model how the backup rewards will be bought. The system should be clear, easy for the child to understand, and should be followed consistently. While the token economy is running, remember to give tokens immediately after a focus behavior is shown. Finally, keep your attention on increasing desired behaviors with rewards/reinforcements, rather than decreasing unwanted behaviors with consequences/ response cost.

To "shut down" a token economy system, consider these six points:

1. First, always pair tokens with encouragement. This will make the transfer from tokens to naturally occurring rewards easier later on.

2. Second, slowly "up the ante," or increase the number of responses needed to get a token. For instance, instead of getting a token for completing one page, make it two pages. This lowers the power of the token.

3.   Third, slowly decrease the time in which the token economy is in effect. For example, it may be in effect all day, every day at first, then cut to half days later on.

4.   Fourth, slowly decrease the availability of backup rewards that are not a part of the natural environment (e.g., movies), and increase the number of items that are (e.g., extra time to play).

5.   Fifth, raise the cost of desirable items (e.g., movies) and lower the cost of less desirable items (favorite snack).

6.   Last, phase out the use of the tokens. For example, gradually shift from using poker chips, to stickers on a paper, to tally marks on a paper, to tally marks kept by the adult.

Considering Contingencies

In this chapter, I shared some tools for helping your child learn that their choices make a difference in what happens next. These tools are rooted in psychology and have been used with success by parents, schools and other institutions. The goal of these tools is to teach children about personal responsibility for their behavior in loving and encouraging ways.

Contingencies provide a way for you to monitor things as your child explores life, learns from it, and grows in their ability to navigate it in healthy and successful ways. It is important for children to learn from their choices in ways that empower them, rather than in ways that take power away from them. We want them to grow up feeling capable, confident, responsible, worthy, and willing to take healthy risks when it's suitable to do so. They will feel these things when:

1.   they experience how their choices can affect their life;

2.   they use their experiences for self-improvement rather than self-punishment or shaming; and

3.   they get loving support and encouragement from the adults in their lives.

5

THERAPY

Teaching new skills for children's
emotional, behavioral, and social thriving

IN MY WORK, I have seen that inattention, over-activity, and impulsivity are often linked to emotional distress or discomfort that a child may be experiencing inside. When people are trying to avoid unpleasant feelings, they tend to "get busy" to distract themselves from the things that really need their attention. Spending time and energy on outside happenings leaves little or no room to focus on the uncomfortable things trying to surface inside.

Calming a child's emotional state inside can free them to focus better on managing their outside behaviors in more healthy ways. As a child's body and mind slow down, feelings they may be trying to avoid can surface. These feelings are often at the root of their behaviors. This is why it is essential to include counseling as a part of the treatment plan for symptoms of a diagnosis such as AD/HD. Emotions that surface as a child's nervous system calms down can best be managed in a therapeutic setting.

Certain types of therapy can be helpful in treating symptoms that are linked specifically to the AD/HD diagnosis. These therapies fit into a holistic model of health care by encouraging children to trust themselves, and to take responsibility for their behavior as a part of their whole system of being in the world. I review a few of the more common types in this chapter, including Dr. Post's Family-Centered Regulatory Therapy, Cognitive-Behavioral Therapy, Play Therapy, and Social Skills Therapy. In addition, you may choose to talk to a school or community psychologist, counselor or therapist about what kinds of services are offered in your area. At the end of the chapter, I provide you with guidelines for choosing a therapy style and a therapist.

Keep in mind that change is a gradual process that cannot be forced. Some behaviors are linked to emotional wounds that may take time to heal before the behavior shifts. This is because sometimes children set up internal behavior patterns out of a perceived need to protect themselves. This patterning will stay in their being as their "default mode" whenever they feel or perceive a threat to their sense of wellbeing or safety. For this patterning to begin to shift, some kids need the safety of a therapeutic setting.

Everyone shifts more readily when they are mentally and emotionally motivated for things to be different, and when they feel that it is safe to make the changes. Trying to force or rush the process of change in kids can create resistance and fear. Some shifts may be seen fairly quickly, but others may take more time and patience. The challenge with this approach is that you must be willing to support your child's healing and growth as it comes over time. The pay-off with this approach is that the changes tend to be more permanent than those provided by other strategies, such as medication.

Dr. Post's Family-Centered Regulatory Therapy

In Chapter 3, I reviewed Dr. Post's stress model of dysregulation, and the *Family-Centered Regulatory Parenting Approach* he developed based on that model. I will not repeat that information here. Instead, in this section, I outline the *Family-Centered Regulatory Therapy* strategy he created as a part of the treatment program for children who are operating in what he calls a state of emotional dysregulation.

Essentially, Dr. Post's approach is linked to family systems theory in psychology, which is based on the idea that each member of a family contributes to the dynamics and functioning of the family as a whole, as well as to the functioning of each individual member. No one family member operates in isolation of the others; their behavior is closely connected. This means that in order to understand and resolve the "problems" that one member may be showing, the other members must be a part of the treatment process.

Along these lines, Dr. Post believes that when a child is in a state of dysregulation, chances are good that the entire family is dysregulated. In his view, family dynamics are considered key to understanding and resolving a child's difficulties. He believes that "the family must be addressed as a unit first, and as individuals second." In his therapy model, he works to bring parents into a state of regulation, or emotional awareness, first, believing that until this happens, there is little hope of achieving regulation within the entire family.

Let's review the basis of his stress model here. Dr. Post believes that behavior is rooted in two things: outside stress and the inside feelings that are triggered by the stress. For example, let's say that at some point in your life, you experienced a stressful event. You might have felt anxious, afraid, sad, humiliated, and the like. These feelings were translated into your behavior, or response to the event. You may have run, screamed, cried, remained silent, and so on. This stress experience was then logged into your biology, or specifically, into your cells. This is called *cellular memory*. Today, scientists have proven that cellular memory exists, so this is no longer theory, but fact.

The problem is that cellular memories are generally held in the unconscious mind, the part that we are not consciously aware of. The emotions that are attached to our cellular memories, then, influence our behavior without us knowing it, and cause us to misinterpret similar situations based on our past experiences. As a result, we may find ourselves over-reacting or responding to events in ways that do not fit the current circumstances because our cellular memory has kicked in and so have our "default coping" patterns.

Remember, the sequence is:
STRESS (Event) $\Rightarrow$ EMOTION (Unconscious, Fear-Based) $\Rightarrow$ BEHAVIOR.

The key to Dr. Post's Regulation Therapy for children is to bring these unconscious emotions to the surface, or into their conscious mind of awareness, so that they can have control over their behavior. In this way, Dr. Post says that children are in a state of *regulation*. On the other hand, when these emotions are not in their conscious awareness (and their behavior is not truly in their control), they are said to be *dysregulated*. Dr. Post believes that this is what happens with many children who are labeled "difficult," such as those diagnosed with AD/HD.

Dr. Post applies this model to parents first, and then to their children. Parents must be regulators of their own emotional states before they can support their children in learning to regulate themselves. Once parents are functioning in a state of regulation, they are taught how to "parent their children toward regulation." In this way, the goal shifts from working with parents on their own regulation, to working with parents on how to maintain regulation in their children. As Dr. Post explained, parents create safety for their child within the parent-child relationship. In this way, parents are able to "teach" regulation to the child. When dysregulated children are repeatedly helped back to a state of regulation by their parents in a positive way, their brains begin to change and develop the ability to self-regulate. Basically, when parents are in a state of regulation, they can provide their children with the support needed to learn how to regulate their own emotions. When children (and adults) are emotionally regulated, they become behaviorally regulated as well (since behavior follows emotion).

In Dr. Post's model, the therapist's role at this stage is to support parents by being available, providing a secure base, and helping them to understand their own unconscious experiences and responses. When the unconscious emotions of parents and children are brought into the conscious mind, they can be "integrated." This results in behavioral responses that are healthier and more aligned with present circumstances instead of past ones, for both parents and children.

Cognitive-Behavioral Therapy

The main focus of "cognitive-behavioral" therapy is to help children become aware of the thoughts that pass through their minds, which, in turn, guide their behavior. By teaching children to pay attention to their thoughts, they can learn to change them and make more successful behavioral choices.

There are five popular types of cognitive-behavioral therapy that can be used with children. They involve a certain amount of self-monitoring and self-management as described in Chapter 4. These include: positive self-talk, self-instruction, thought stopping, visualization or imagery, and problem solving strategies.

Positive self-talk is when children are taught to say positive and encouraging things to themselves while doing challenging tasks. For example, "You can do it! Keep trying. You are doing great!" In this way, kids learn to be their own cheerleaders and to keep their focus on what they are doing. By learning to say positive, supportive things to themselves, children can lower their frustration levels and keep from getting too discouraged or overwhelmed by a task.

With *self-instruction,* which is closely related to positive self-talk, children learn to give themselves mental reminders about what to do and what not to do: "Keep your hands to yourself in the hall. Walk in single file. No talking." In this way, they begin to manage their own behaviors. These two techniques generally start out with the talk being spoken aloud, and then shift to a whisper, and eventually to silence (within their own mind). In this way, the therapist and other adults can coach a child in using the techniques when needed, before they begin to do it on their own.

Thought stopping is similar to positive self-talk and self-instruction. With thought stopping, children are literally taught to interrupt negative or inappropriate streams of thought, and shift them to something more positive and appropriate. For example, when a child becomes aware that they are thinking, "This is too hard. I will never be able to finish it on time," they can stop those negative thoughts and consciously replace them with positive ones. They may replace them with something like, "I can do this. I can ask for help. I can get it done on time." With this method, children can also learn to identify and correct any errors in their thinking, such as if they have misinterpreted an event or made a false assumption. Problem solving strategies can be added as well (like the ones reviewed in Chapter 3 or below), to make this a powerful technique and life skill for children.

Visualization or *imagery* is another cognitive-behavioral strategy that is used with children. This is reviewed again in Chapter 7 under "Relaxation Using The Mind." In the context of cognitive-behavioral therapy, children learn to picture something in their mind's eye. Depending on what their challenge is, they can either envision something negative whenever they get the urge to misbehave, or they can envision something positive whenever they are tense. In psychology, this is known as "covert conditioning:" by pairing an image with an urge, the urge will eventually take on the feelings created by the image. Ultimately, the urge alone will trigger the feelings. When this pairing of image with urge is repeated many times until the urge alone creates the feelings, covert conditioning has taken place. The urge has been "conditioned" to create a certain feeling. For example, if every time a child got the urge to curse, they imagined their mother washing their mouth out with icky soap, the urge alone would eventually stir up negative feelings, and the cursing behavior would diminish over time. On the other hand, if a child with a fear of planes visualized them floating on the wings of sweet guardian angels every time they saw one, the fear should eventually decrease.

Visualization can also be used to boost a child's confidence about something by having them picture the event with a positive outcome. For instance, a child who is nervous about an upcoming test can repeatedly envision themselves entering the testing room and sitting down calmly; feeling completely confident and ready; taking the test without a hitch; feeling good about it; and seeing an "A" on the top of their graded test paper. Of course, the actual process is more involved than I am presenting here, but you get the idea. It is a fact that many famous athletes use this technique before they compete.

Problem solving is also considered a cognitive-behavioral strategy, since it involves both thoughts and actions. There are many examples out there that provide the kind of structure that is useful and helpful with children who are impulsive, inattentive, distractible, and hyperactive. These techniques break tasks into smaller steps, help them organize their thoughts, and cue them to remember the steps by using an acronym. Most children can learn them with practice.

Here is an example of a problem-solving strategy that I created for children that is especially useful with impulsive behavior. I kept it simple and easy to remember. If a child is in a situation where they are having a lot of emotion around a situation, it's helpful to acknowledge and validate what they are feeling first, either before moving into a problem-solving strategy or perhaps using a problem-solving strategy. This one is similar to the thought-stopping technique, but is more for behaviors. I call it *STOP*:

S - stop what you are doing,
T - think about the end (result),
O - open (your mind) to other choices;
P - pick a safe (or kind, friendly, loving) one to try instead.

With this strategy, children learn to tell themselves to STOP (as in thought-stopping), which is also the first step of many problem-solving processes. This accomplishes several things. First, the use of the acronym STOP makes it easy for them to remember. Second, stopping is generally a good first step in situations of conflict or danger anyway. Third, the word "stop" can cue their brains to the other three steps in this strategy, whether they say it or someone else does. Fourth, once they stop, they are in a better position to move on to the next step(s). Fifth, stopping is something that they can learn to do themselves. And finally, since stopping is generally something they can master fairly quickly, they will feel some success with the strategy early in the process of learning it. This will motivate them to keep trying until they master all the steps.

Cognitive-behavioral therapies are effective in teaching children some tools they can use to manage and shift their own behavior. Research shows that for some, but not all children, these techniques make a very positive difference for symptoms of inattention, impulsivity, and hyperactivity. There are also the added benefits of taking responsibility for their own behavior, feeling self-pride when they are successful, and getting positive feedback from important adults around them. In this way, their sense of self-esteem will also be nourished.

Play therapy

Dr. Virginia M. Axline, an expert in the area of play therapy and credited with developing the non-directive model, wrote that "Play therapy is based upon the fact that play is the child's natural medium of self-expression. It is an opportunity which is given to the child to 'play out' his feelings and problems just as, in certain types of adult therapy, an individual 'talks out' his difficulties."[3]

Play therapy is a well-researched technique that allows children to work through their inner conflicts through play. During play therapy, children heal, learn and grow through symbolic play, and through linking the symbolism to real-life situations. Play is one way that children communicate with others. Play therapy is a wonderful way to work with children because it gives them a safe way to express their feelings when they cannot find the right words.

Play is a very natural and fun thing for children to do, so there is usually no resistance to the therapy. Play therapy works like this: the conflicts that children feel inside show up in their play with toys, objects, or with other children. When the feelings appear, the therapist can work with the child through the play to understand and express them in healthy ways. The therapist may decide to move the issues from the symbolic level of play, to the realistic level of the child's life. This transfer, however, is not necessary for play therapy to be effective. It will work through the symbology of the play alone.

There are two models of play therapy, each with its own purpose. In the first, known as *directive play therapy*, the therapist takes an active role in the session, assuming responsibility for guiding and interpreting the play. Directive play therapy can be useful in situations where it would be helpful for a child to learn specific social skills, for example. In these instances, the play therapy situation can be used by the therapist to symbolically model certain skills for the child. Then, the therapist can gradually transfer the skills from the symbolic level to real life situations for the child. The therapist might have the child identify when certain skills might be useful in real life, and have them practice the skills in the session.

In the second, called, *non-directive play therapy*, the therapist gives control of the session to the child, allowing them to guide and direct the play. The therapist maintains an active role in the session, but under the child's leadership, in the position of being a mirror to clarify and reflect what they express. This model is based on the idea that children have everything they need within themselves to grow into healthy, happy adults. They are, by nature, completely okay and lovable beings.

What non-directive play therapy provides children is a safe place (physically and emotionally) to be themselves, to express their true natures, to get to know and accept themselves, and to make whatever changes they choose to in the direction of creating a more satisfying "blueprint of life" for themselves. There is no judgment, no pressure to change, no control over – nothing that will leave the child feeling that they are not good enough, smart enough, capable enough, lovable enough, etc. They are simply given an opportunity to show who they are, explore any unconscious ideas, discover their potentials, and shoot for the stars, if they choose to, with the understanding that whatever they are and whatever they choose is okay in that setting. The therapist serves as a safe and nonjudgmental "mirror" for them, so they can take a clear look at themselves. There are certain boundaries that the play therapist will maintain for safety reasons, but other than this, children are free to choose, and then learn from their choices.

Through play therapy, children can learn and practice important life skills like creative thinking, the power of choice and the results of their choices, how to deal with conflicts with others, problem-solving, cooperation, teamwork, leadership, and self-confidence. They can also learn about trust, empathy, respect, sharing and kindness. They get a feel for the role of social rules, taking risks, respecting limits, and the difference between fantasy and reality. And the play therapy setting gives them a safe place to practice the new skills. The goal is for children to transfer what they learn in the play therapy room to the world outside.

Research shows that play therapy is an effective way to deal with children's social, emotional, behavioral, and learning challenges, including the symptoms of AD/HD, stress and trauma, anxiety, depression, aggression, conduct problems, low self-esteem, reading difficulties, and social skills problems. Research also shows that it takes an average of twenty sessions to resolve a child's issues, though this will vary depending on severity. In my experience, play (including art) therapy is one of the most effective strategies to use with children, including those in pre-kindergarten through high school. They respond well to it, are motivated to participate, and usually, positive changes can be seen shortly after the therapy begins.

Social Skills Therapy

Being a socially skilled person is important in life. Socially skilled children are able to make and keep friends, introduce themselves to new people, cooperate, and compromise. They are comfortable in new situations, and are trusting and trustworthy. They are conflict-managers, respectful of differences, assertive rather than aggressive, willing to admit to mistakes, and willing to stand up for what they believe in. They are also at lower risk for developing emotional difficulties related to depression, anxiety, and low self-esteem. They grow into well-adjusted adults.

Children with behaviors such as impulsivity, distractibility, anxiety, over-excitability, shyness, bossiness, withdrawal, and aggression can benefit from learning how to interact with others in more successful ways. Behaviors such as impulsivity and hyperactivity can interfere with their ability to make lasting friendships with their peers. Sometimes children are so nervous about "fitting in," being accepted and liked, or being embarrassed or teased, that they behave strangely or in ways that are not okay to others. Their social behavior may be so different from the expectations of their peers that they are alienated or feel socially isolated.

In social skills therapy, children become aware of how they relate to others, and learn to fine-tune their social behaviors. The main goals of social skills therapy are to teach children to notice and respond appropriately to social cues, or signals, from others; to learn healthy ways to express their feelings; to respect feelings shown by others; and to speak with more confidence. Many of the skills taught to children are the same skills we reviewed earlier in the parenting section for parents, such as problem solving, using "I-messages," making eye contact, speaking clearly, and acknowledging feelings.

Social skills therapy can include things like cooperative game play, group projects or activities, modeling and role-play, guided practice, behavioral rehearsal, feedback, videotapes, problem solving, weekly lessons, or one-on-one coaching and practice. As with other skills, social skills may come more naturally for some, but must be learned and practiced by others. When children learn social coping skills, they become more comfortable around others and can treat them more kindly. Part of what is gained is a stronger sense of self-worth, self-esteem, and confidence. A strong sense of self goes a long way toward forming healthy relationships with others. Social skills training has been shown to help children manage their behavior. For children diagnosed with AD/HD, research shows that a combination of treatments, including behavioral management, social skills training, and for some, medication, produces more positive and lasting improvements than any treatment alone.

Guidelines For Selecting a Therapy And Therapist

As you may have noticed in reading this chapter, many of the skills and strategies overlap in their content. This makes them very compatible with each other. Many of the strategies can be used together or as a bridge from one to another. These are skills and strategies that can be taught through a school by the psychologist or counselor, or at a private agency that offers children's therapies. Parents can also learn these strategies from a therapist or counselor, and then teach them to their children. Here are some suggestions for choosing which method to use:

1. Select a therapist or counselor the way you would select the ideal caregiver for your child: Get referrals from people you know and trust. If you'd like, you can get the professional license number of the therapist or counselor and call their licensing board to be sure no complaints have been filed against them. Have a phone or face-to-face consultation with each candidate to discuss their methods, beliefs, philosophies, ethics, background, etc., so that you get an idea of who they are, what they stand for, and how they approach therapy. Make sure that their approach and beliefs are comfortable to you and in line with your own. Clarify that you are willing to be a partner in the process, and be prepared to be on your child's "therapeutic team." This will be your best bet at getting positive results for your child.

Do not be afraid to ask them questions or express any concerns you may have about the situation. Do not be afraid to talk to them about any wishes you may have to change plans once they start working with your child. This is your right as the parent. Be certain, however, that any change is handled in a way that is not traumatic to your child, so that your child has a chance to experience a healthy ending with the therapist or counselor if the relationship is going to end suddenly.

2. Select the best type of therapy for your child: Successful therapy for adults is very different from successful therapy for children and adolescents. Research shows that for children and adolescents, "talk therapy" usually doesn't work. Choose a therapist who will not expect your child to behave like a "little adult" in their office. Instead, select a professional who is trained as a play therapist, art therapist, movement or music therapist who can provide something that is aligned with your youngster's needs, interests and ability level. Make certain that the therapist has experience in working with children who have the types of issues that seem to be bothering your child. Otherwise, you may end up disappointed.

3. Consider using a therapist or counselor as a coach to you: This way, you can learn to support your child in mastering new skills for handling their social relationships, emotional expression, and behavior. Teaching children in the familiar settings in which they live makes it easier for them to generalize the skills to different situations. This also puts you in the position of being on hand and "in the know" to support their efforts, and to consult with school personnel in doing the same.

4. Consider setting something up through your child's school: These days, parents and school personnel are partners in nurturing children's social and emotional wellbeing. Many schools have programs for students that address social skills, behavior management, and emotional growth. If your child is not already participating, consider checking with the school psychologist or counselor to see what programs are available to your child, and when they could attend. You might also consider consulting with the school psychologist or counselor about your child's behavior and developing a coaching relationship with them, if they are able to provide one. The benefit of this type of relationship with the school is that it is free of charge to you, and school personnel are available to your child and you on a daily basis.

The drawback to this type of situation is that school psychologists and counselors are limited in what they can offer to children and especially their parents, due to the high demands of their job and limitations within the school setting. The schools are not mandated or resourced to serve as long-term therapy clinics for children and their families. Instead, they are set up to focus on short-term issues that relate specifically to children's ability to succeed in school, such as enhancing social and behavioral skills at school. Beyond that, the school setting may not be the best match for serving your child's therapy needs, and you may choose to take them to a private clinic if more intensive therapy is called for.

6

NUTRITION

How it is linked to children's health,
moods, and behavior

IN TODAY'S WORLD, we hear a lot of talk about nutrition and kids' weight, yet we don't hear much about nutrition and kids' behavior. Why is that, when there is plenty of research documenting the link between what kids put into their bellies and what happens to their brains and behavior as a result? Did you know that there is a direct link between the belly and the brain? This is why adults drink caffeinated beverages in the mornings to "wake up" and why people get sleepy after eating something with a lot of sugar or carbohydrates (which turn to sugar in the body). Certain substances can affect a person's moods and behavior within as little as one minute, particularly if they have a sensitivity to it. This is how the body works. So it's no surprise to know that the things kids eat and drink have a direct impact on not only their health, but on their brains, their moods, and their behavior.

That is why one of the more popular ways of dealing with hyperactivity, impulsivity and inattention using a holistic health model has been to work with nutrition. The Center for Science in the Public Interest published a report in 1999 alleging that government agencies, physicians and the food industry have all chosen to ignore strong evidence that nutrition is linked to hyperactivity. It is interesting to note that there are a lot of published books and research articles supporting the link between nutrition and the symptoms of AD/HD that are not talked about much. As far back as 1982, the National Institutes of Health (NIH) held a conference to review the research results on the link between diet and hyperactivity. The panel found that there *was* a drop in hyperactivity as a result of changes in the diet. They recommended that more research be done on the diet-behavior connection. Now that the research results are in, there is *no question* that nutrition *is* linked to many of the symptoms we call AD/HD. Read on…

The Scoop About Nutrition: What The Research Shows

What research shows today is that a healthy diet chosen specifically for a person's own needs *does* get rid of the symptoms of AD/HD for many children and adults. Nutrition *does* make a difference. We have known for some time that nutrition makes a big difference in our general state of health, for example, by strengthening our bodies' ability to fight off illnesses and recover from injuries. We also know that nutrition and a healthy lifestyle make a positive difference in our state of mind, in our ability to handle stress, and in the way we choose to behave every day. So, besides being a good way to prevent health problems and extend a person's life, proper nutrition can be a natural and gentle way to deal with the symptoms of AD/HD for many people.

Experts who study AD/HD are beginning to consider it a neuro-metabolic issue. For example, Dr. Titus Venessa, a research scientist, author, and Founder and President of Forever Young Health Foods in Central Florida, claims that neuro-metabolic dysfunction interferes with the development of neural connections, neuronal density, and neurotransmitter production, which then directly affects our behavior. Basically, a neuro-metabolic dysfunction means that there is a disorder in the central nervous system, which relates to attention, concentration, learning, memory and information processing. Neuro-metabolic functioning is directly linked to what kinds of food we eat, and how the food is converted by our metabolism. The body's metabolic process converts the food into usable energy for cell and brain activity. So, what we eat each day *directly* influences our mental and behavioral functioning.

Along these lines, there is plenty of evidence in the research showing that nutrition and diet are linked to the symptoms of AD/HD. The most common food ingredients or chemicals that cause a physical, behavioral, and/or emotional reaction in children are:

1. artificial flavorings (e.g., monosodium glutamate, or MSG);

2. artificial colorings (e.g., FD&C No...; Yellow #5 & 10; Blue #1 & 2; Red #1, 2, & 3; Green #3; "Color Added");

3. artificial preservatives (e.g., Butylated Hydroxyanisole, or BHA; Butylated Hydroxytoluene, or BHT; Tertiary Butyl-hydroquinone, or TBHQ; Sorbic Acid; Nitrites and Nitrates; Sulfites; Sodium Benzoate; Benzoic Acid);

4. sugars and sugar substitutes (e.g., white, brown, or cane sugar; corn syrup, high fructose corn syrup, and brown rice syrup - which are different names for sugar; NutraSweet, Aspartame, Equal, Saccharin, Sweet 'n Low, and Sucralose); and

5. caffeine.

This is a partial list. An additional list can be found on page 109, under "Additional Findings About Nutrition and Diet." Other nutritional issues that can lead to physical, behavioral, and/or emotional reactions in children include:

1. diets containing too much yeast;
2. diets containing too little vitamins, minerals, or amino acids;
3. diets that result in overacidity of the body; and
4. lead or aluminum poisoning.

Food sensitivities or allergies are also known to cause physical, behavioral, and emotional reactions, including symptoms such as hyperactivity, oppositional-defiance, depression, irritability, weight gain, chronic ear infections, and bedwetting. For example, Dr. Arturo M. Volpe, Doctor of Chiropractic, Certified Clinical Nutritionist, and Fellow of the International Academy of Medical Acupuncture, claims that gluten, which is a protein found in certain grains, has been found to cause severe reactions in some children. Gluten sensitivity or intolerance can result in a life-threatening disease called, Celiac Disease, and has also been linked to such disorders as autism and AD/HD.

Likewise, Dr. Volpe maintains that high amounts of starch from foods made with refined grains (such as breads, pastas, pizza dough, cereals, and cookies), and even from potatoes and corn (which are starchy foods), often cause allergic reactions. Too much starch in the diet can result in hyperactivity, a weakened immune system, and nutritional deficiencies. It can take up to three days for a food to make its way through the body, and some substances or chemicals can stay in the body for months. That is why these allergies are often referred to as a "delayed food sensitivity," because it can be several hours, or even days, before a reaction shows up after eating the "trigger" food. They are also referred to as "hidden food allergies," because when the reaction is from a food that is eaten on a daily basis, it can be hard to identify the culprit.

As further evidence of the link between nutrition and children's functioning, consider these research findings from studies done with children diagnosed as having AD/HD:

1. Kids who responded to the Feingold Diet had much higher amounts of copper in their bodies than kids who did not respond to the diet (See more information on the Feingold Diet on page 108 under "Additional Findings About Nutrition and Diet);

2. Kids who were given a "nutrient dense diet" in 813 state facilities showed great improvements in their conduct, intelligence, and/or academic performance;

3. A review of the research shows that diet greatly affects the behavior of most children, as do some non-food items like perfumes, toxic fumes, or inhalants;

4. Kids who were fed certain "reactive foods" (after having not eaten the foods for a time) had unusually more betal brain-wave activity in certain areas of their brains after eating the foods; this means that the foods kicked certain parts of their brains into "fast motion;"

5. When kids were not allowed to eat certain "reactive foods" and foods with artificial colors, 73% had positive behavior changes;

6. One research review shows that (a) synthetic food colors and food dyes have negative effects on learning, behavior, and the way the body works; (b) taking certain foods out of the diet controls behavior in cases of AD/HD in anywhere from 58% to 82% of the cases; and (c) vitamin B6 worked better than Ritalin for the treatment of hyperactivity in a small study, both in amount of improvement and how long it lasted after stopping the treatment.

7. Magnesium deficiency, frequent use of antibiotics (resulting in a weakened immune system and overgrowth of yeast organisms or fungal metabolites), and below average amounts of essential fatty acids in children have all been linked to the symptoms linked to the AD/HD diagnosis.

These research findings, which span from the 1970s through the 1990s, begin to give us a glimpse of how important nutrition is in the AD/HD issue. The rest of this chapter covers other findings that further support the connection between nutrition and the symptoms of AD/HD in children.

Additional Findings About Nutrition And Diet

The famous "Feingold Diet," which was developed and promoted by Dr. Benjamin Feingold in 1975, was the first of its kind. Dr. Feingold felt that at least half of the children seen as hyperactive, impulsive, and inattentive were reacting to additives in their food. His diet cuts out additives, artificial flavorings, food colorings, and preservatives. Although the diet takes some effort to carry out at first, research shows that it does work wonderfully for some children diagnosed with AD/HD (despite what is reported in some sources).

I have found that making the food buying changes takes some time initially, but then becomes easy, once you know what products you want and like. With all of the whole food, organic markets and products springing up these days, it is fairly easy to find what you are looking for in one shopping trip. It is important to read labels when you first start this process, and educate yourself as to what the labels mean. Most products today are clearly marked with, for example, "no sugar added," "no artificial sweeteners," "organically grown," "no artificial preservatives," and "gluten/wheat free." Be aware that some companies have found ways to label items that may sound good, but really are not what you want. For instance, "corn syrup" and "high fructose corn syrup" are sugar, and "all natural" can mean any number of things. Evaporated Cane Sugar is, after all, "all natural," but it is still added sugar in the food. Stevia is a natural plant sweetener that does not seem to affect mood and behavior, so is a good sugar substitute.

Several food additives have been identified that can account for damage and irritation to the nervous system in children, as well as overactivity, difficulty sleeping, tendency for accidents, etc. The following list comes from David Hoffmann's 1988 book, *The Herbal Handbook* and includes well-known culprits, although the complete list is much longer. These should be avoided as much as possible. The law requires that packages be labeled as containing these additives, so if food packages are not clearly labeled, there is usually a toll-free phone number to call or an address to write with questions:

E102 (Tartrazine)	E133 (Brilliant Blue)
E104 (Quinoline Yellow)	E150 (Caramel)
E107 (Yellow 2G)	E151 (Black PN)
E110 (Sunset Yellow)	E154 (Brown FK)
E120 (Cochineal)	E155 (Brown HT)
E122 (Carmoisine)	E210 (Benzoic Acid)
E123 (Amaranth)	E211 (Sodium Benzoate)
E124 (Ponceau 4R)	E250 (Sodium Nitrite)
E127 (Erythosine)	E251 (Sodium Nitrate)
E128 (Red 2G)	E320 (Butylated Hydroxyanisole)
E132 (Indigo Carmine)	E321 (Butylated Hydroxytoluene)

Dr. Leo Galland, a holistic physician in New York City and author of *Super Immunity for Kids*, is worried about how unhealthy the average American diet has gotten in the past 50 years. It is a well-known fact that the neurotransmitters that control our brains need a steady supply of nutrients to work right. When our intake of nutrients is out of balance, it can affect our behavior. In general, the food we eat today has become overly processed and "underly" nutritious. It contains too much sugar and refined carbohydrates, and too little of what our brains need like vitamins, minerals, and fatty acids. Food sensitivities or allergies can also affect our brains and nervous system, keeping them from working properly. The most common sensitivities or allergies are to milk, wheat, corn, yeast, soy, and food additives. Dr. Galland gives suggestions for ways to help the brain, nervous system, and body stay in the nutritional balance that it needs to grow and work right. This book is a great resource for interested parents.

Another good resource about the link between diet and AD/HD is a booklet written by Nina Anderson and Dr. Howard Peiper entitled, *A.D.D.: The Natural Approach*. They detail how nutrition, trace minerals, magnesium, zinc, enzymes, essential fatty acids, proanthcyanidins (antioxidants), and dimethylglycine supplement (DMG) affect the body's ability to work right. These authors note that "placing a child on a natural organic foods diet will help the body rid itself of toxins and restore the right vitamins, minerals, and other nutrients to the brain."[4] This is good advice for general health and wellbeing, and can be helpful when dealing with symptoms of AD/HD.

Susan Stockton, MA, CRC, has written several health books and health articles for newspapers and magazines. She has also spent more than a decade both teaching and studying alternative health care, and providing counseling and adult education about health and drugs, both publicly and privately. In her booklet, *ADD: Drug-Free Alternatives for Hyperactivity & Aggression*, she very clearly presents research on how symptoms of AD/HD are linked to diet, including food additives, allergies, yeast, sugar, lead, minerals, overall nutritional deficiency, over-acidity, and amino acids. The idea is that an imbalance in any of these things can keep the body's systems from working in harmony, which can lead to hyperactivity, impulsivity, inattention, and other challenging behaviors. Dietary changes will not only improve AD/HD symptoms, but will strengthen the overall ability of the body to work in a healthful way. Stockton reports on the success of many doctors who remove unhealthy foods and food ingredients from children's diets, and begin a nutritionally balanced dietary program for them. Her book is a very useful resource for people who are interested in the dietary connection.

Along these lines, author Laura Stevens wrote a book entitled, *12 Effective Ways to Help Your ADD/ADHD Child*, in which she thoroughly reviews AD/HD, possible causes, prevention ideas, and 12 ways to help that include mostly dietary and nutritional changes. Stevens has studied the role of nutrition and food sensitivities in AD/HD for over 20 years, and is considered a pioneer in this area. The research she reviewed shows that changes in diet and nutrition *do* have successful results for many children. She includes a chapter on how to help your child adjust to a new diet with tips for shopping, cooking, holidays, and some tasty recipes to use. Her book is another great resource for parents who are serious about working with their child's diet and nutrition for handling the symptoms of AD/HD.

Dr. Volpe, who I mentioned earlier in relation to food allergies and sensitivities, strongly believes that natural and homeopathic treatments (including diet and nutrition) *do* make a positive difference for children and adults dealing with various physical, emotional, and behavioral symptoms. He highlights the link between the brain and the stomach as the most important bodily connection, since what we eat feeds the neurotransmitters in the brain and keeps them working correctly. In fact, research shows that the cells in the brain and the cells in the stomach "talk" directly to each other to try to keep the body's systems working and in balance. Without a healthy diet and good nutrition, the neurotransmitters and other parts of the brain begin to "act up." Since the brain is the organ that controls *all* of our bodily functions, when it is not properly fed, reactions show up in our physical and mental states, emotions, behavior, and energy. By keeping our brains healthy and properly fed, we keep our entire body healthy and working smoothly. This translates into balance within our physical, mental, emotional, and energetic states of being.

Dr. Volpe has found that lowering the intake of sugar, caffeine, food dyes, and carbohydrates, for example, and balancing the amounts of fatty and amino acids in the body, are some of the main ways to obtain a decrease in symptoms linked to a diagnosis of AD/HD. Not only do things like sugar and caffeine add to problems with our general health, but eating them usually creates a cycle of physical, mental, emotional, and energetic "ups and downs" in which there is an initial "rush" of energy that is followed by a hard "fall" in energy shortly afterwards. They also *absorb* important nutrients from the body on their way through, creating a "double whammy" effect.

In Dr. Volpe's experience, children and adults with symptoms linked to the AD/HD diagnosis have had great and lasting success with changes in diet and nutrition *that are specifically chosen for their unique needs.* He claims that for most people, improvements are seen and felt in three to four weeks. These are very startling and impressive results! Aside from diet and nutrition, Dr. Volpe's treatments for the symptoms linked to AD/HD often include relaxation and stress management (discussed in Chapter 7), CranioSacral and acupuncture therapies (discussed in Chapter 9), and the use of a special hyperbaric (oxygen) chamber.

Nutritional Supplements

Many professionals suggest that nutritional supplements are effective treatments for behavioral issues in some individuals. Studies have found a link between behavior and deficiencies in certain minerals such as zinc, calcium and magnesium. Other nutritionists recommend supplementing the B vitamins (Thiamin [B1], Riboflavin [B2], Niacin, Pyridoxine [B6], Folic acid, and B12), and vitamins C and E. *A trained clinical nutritionist, however, must manage this treatment approach, since each person's needs are different.* Taking too high a dosage of vitamins and minerals can be harmful to the body. For example, vitamins A and D, and the mineral selenium, are toxic or poisonous to the body in large amounts. There are also reports that large or mega-doses of certain vitamins can make symptoms worse for some hyperactive children.

Keep in mind that manufactured vitamins and minerals cannot substitute for good nutrition obtained from natural food sources. Our bodies absorb nutrients from pills or other manufactured sources differently than how they absorb nutrients from natural food sources. So, do not make the mistake of thinking that you can shortcut good nutrition by using mega-doses of vitamins or minerals.

In their book, *Let's Play Doctor*, Drs. J.D. Wallach, a veterinarian and naturopathic physician, and Ma Lan, a medical doctor, among others, identified a number of symptoms that are linked with certain nutritional deficiencies. A few of the symptoms related to AD/HD, and their correlating nutritional deficiencies, are listed in the table below for you to consider:

Symptom	Deficiency
Hyperactivity, Restlessness	Calcium, Copper, Essential Fatty Acids (Omega-3, Omega-6)
Inattention, Cognitive Impairment, Confusion, Memory Loss	Magnesium, Potassium, Sodium, Zinc
Anxiety, Nervousness	Chromium, Magnesium, Vitamin B-1 (Thiamin)
Depression, Fatigue, Irritability, Apathy, Crying Spells, Moodiness, Tiredness	Calcium; Chromium; Copper; Sodium; Magnesium; Potassium; Vitamins C, B-1 (Thiamin), B-6 (Pyridoxine), B-12; Zinc
Coordination Impairment	Vitamin B-1 (Thiamin)

Not surprisingly, nutritional supplement products are being aggressively marketed on the Internet, TV, radio, and in magazines today for various illnesses, conditions, and symptoms. An example of one such product directed at the symptoms linked to AD/HD (for adults) is "Pycnogenol," which was invented in France by Jack Masquelier. This product was recently made available in the U.S. as MASQUELIER'S® due to some unresolved trademark issues with the name Pycnogenol. It is a powerful antioxidant nutritional compound that is derived from maritime pine bark and grape seed extract, creating a special blend of bioflavonoids. MASQUELIER'S® is described as a 100% non-toxic, natural, non-drug nutritional supplement. It is said to be much more effective than vitamin E, has the same health effects of vitamin C, and "protects brain and nerve tissue with its unique ability to penetrate the blood-brain barrier."

MASQUELIER'S® is now patented as a natural extract in the U.S. for treating a diagnosis of AD/HD (U.S. Patent # 5,719,178) and is being recommended by some progressive doctors for this purpose, primarily with adults. It does not yet have the approval of the US Food and Drug Administration (FDA). Remember that supplements like Pycnogenol are not meant to substitute for proper nutrition from whole food sources. Supplements may support the body's overall activities, but as we have seen, there is no "magic pill" that can make specific issues disappear. As with any treatment, Pycnogenol may not work for everybody; its beneficial and side effects will vary according to an individual's unique profile. *It is advisable to consult a holistic doctor, naturopath or pediatrician before using any supplemental product for your child.*

Studies that are currently underway on the link between Pycnogenol and the specific symptoms linked to the AD/HD diagnosis show some promising yet mixed results, so more research is needed. Basically, research is showing that symptoms may dramatically decrease with Pycnogenol because it helps the brain communicate more harmoniously with the body's immune system, improves circulation to the brain, and helps deliver nutrients to the brain.

Early research also suggests that it may support the enzymes that help regulate dopamine and norepinephrine, two of the brain's main neurotransmitters. I believe that similar results can be achieved, however, with the use of a healthy, organic, well-balanced, whole-foods diet. The body and brain are set up to function perfectly on their own (barring injury), when fed the proper nutrition. With a healthy diet, supplements like Pycnogenol may not be needed for the brain and body to work harmoniously together.

There are some reported side effects with Pycnogenol, such as stomach irritation, nausea, flatulence, constipation, acute abdominal pain, and bloating. There have been rare cases of more severe side effects, including kidney stones, hypercalcimia and anorexia. Additionally, it may interfere with the body's use of certain vitamins and minerals, and may clash with certain chemicals in other medications. All of these issues are why it is so important to work with a knowledgeable holistic doctor before using any kind of nutritional supplement, rather than assuming that it is a good match for your unique child.

Another supplement that is marketed as safe and formulated by doctors for the treatment of AD/HD-like symptoms is called ATTEND, by Vaxa. On its website, Vaxa claims that this supplement "supplies the nutrients associated with learning and concentration" that "support the body's natural ability to:

- help calm and reduce stress and frustration;
- help focus attention and increase concentration;
- allow smooth, balanced information processing;
- flush toxins, plaque, and free radicals from brain pathways; and
- increase the flow of nutrients, oxygen, and energy to the brain."

They also claim that it is all natural, has no side effects, and contains no drugs. The website lists the ingredients, of which most are recognizable, such as fatty acids, essential amino acids, flax seed powder, ginkgo biloba, gotukola, pycnogenol, white pine bark, and micronutrients. This product comes with a 30-day, money back guarantee. I have not worked with this product, and do not know anything more about it. I could not find any information about this product listed with the FDA or with reliable online medical resources. As with any supplement, I suggest that you check with a reputable naturopath, holistic doctor, or with your pediatrician before trying it.

The Nutritional Food Guide Pyramid

The U.S. Department of Agriculture (USDA) developed the "Food Guide Pyramid" in 1992 to serve as a blueprint for a healthy American diet. Although it has been changed over the years, the basics have stayed the same. The Guide encourages a diet that includes a variety of foods and low amounts of fat. Basically, it supports a diet consisting mostly of grains (such as whole-grain breads, cereals, rice, pasta); fruits, and vegetables; some dairy (such as milk, yogart, and cheeses) and protein sources (such as lean meats, poultry, fish, beans, eggs, and nuts); and very little fats and sugars (soft drinks, candy, desserts). You can access the Guide online at www.MyPyramid.gov. There is a different version of the Guide for kids and adults, since growing children have slightly different nutritional needs than adults.

Basically, the USDA recommends that for a 1,800-calorie daily diet, kids need:

- 6 ounces of whole grains
- 2 ½ cups of (fresh or lightly cooked) vegetables
- 1 ½ cups of (fresh, unsweetened) fruits
- 3 cups of milk or dairy foods for calcium
- 5 ounces of lean meats and beans for protein
- Oils are not a food group, yet some amounts of them are healthy; get them from things like fish, nuts, and healthy liquid plant-based oils such as olive, soy, or coconut.

Focusing on these food groups and amounts creates a well-balanced diet with variety, fiber, and nutrition to support children's energy and growth. According to the USDA's nutritional guide for children around five years of age, one serving could include any of the following (younger children need fewer servings; older children need more):

Grains
1 slice of bread, tortilla, roll, pancake, biscuit, or waffle
½ cup cooked cereal, rice, or pasta
4 small square saltine crackers
2 small square graham crackers
¾ cup ready-to-eat cereal

Vegetables and Fruits
¼ cup cooked or canned vegetable or fruit
½ piece raw vegetable or fruit
¼ cup fruit or tomato juice

Meat, Poultry, Fish, Dry Beans, Eggs & Nuts
2 oz. cooked lean beef, turkey, chicken, fish, or pork
3 Tbsp. peanut butter
½ cup dried beans or peas
1 egg

1 ½ wieners cut into fourths, lengthwise
1 ½ slices lunch meat/cold cuts

Milk, Yogurt & Cheese
6 oz. low-fat milk
1 oz. low-fat cheese
1 cup cottage cheese
¾ cup low-fat yogurt
¾ cup pudding, custard, or flan (made with low-fat milk)
1 cup soup made with low-fat milk
1 cup ice milk or frozen yogurt

From my own research, I would consider increasing the amount of raw or lightly cooked vegetables; raw, non-dried, and non-sugared fruits; and non-meat protein sources in the diet (such as nuts, seeds, peas, beans, and high-protein grains like quinoa). Ideally, look for "whole" grain products; organic nuts, fruits, and vegetables; meats and dairy products without hormones or chemicals; and use fresh or frozen fruits and vegetables rather than canned when possible (fresh and frozen produce maintains more of its nutritional value than canned tends to).

There are several different versions of food guides available and based on the USDA's version, mostly created by nutrition experts and researchers. In my opinion, Dr. Walter C. Willett, MD, Chair of the Department of Nutrition at the Harvard School of Public Health, has one of the most balanced models based on current research. His food pyramid first appeared in his book *Eat, Drink, and Be Healthy* published by Simon and Schuster in 2001, and is continually being updated according to the latest research findings in nutrition and health. The original pyramid he developed is geared toward adults, yet Dr. Willett and his Harvard team are conducting research for a children's version. You can access the Harvard School of Public Health's Department of Nutrition Web site, The Nutrition Source, at www. hsph.harvard.edu.nutritionsource/. This site is packed with current, research-based information on nutrition, diet, and health.

Food Guides can help you begin to view your family's eating patterns in a new, healthier way than you may have in the past. Keep in mind that the easiest way to make dietary changes is one small step at a time. Consider introducing changes in your family's diet slowly and steadily. Make one change per week and see what happens when you stick with it. Simply replacing sodas and sweets with alternatives like water, tea, nuts, cheeses, and fruits, for example, can make a significant difference. You might be surprised at how different you and your family will feel and behave after eating less sugar and fat, and more grains, fruits, and vegetables for a few weeks. Remember, a healthy body inside means a healthy person outside.

A Word About Food Storage

Although I have not seen any studies linking the chemicals in certain food storage containers to children's behavior, there is growing evidence that links them to things like cancers and abnormal development in animals. Plastic cling wrap, Styrofoam, plastic cartons, plastic bottles, and plastic bags are a primary way that our society has packaged and stored food for years. Not only is this questionable from a health standpoint, but plastics take a very, very long time to biodegrade in our landfills, and when they do, they leach toxic chemicals into the food chain.

PVC (polyvinyl chloride, or vinyl) is a type of plastic used in cling wraps and other food storage containers. When PVC plastics are manufactured and incinerated, dioxins are released into the air and water, which then go into the food chain and eventually make their way into our own fatty tissues through the meat and dairy products we eat. These plastic food containers also leach questionable chemicals directly into the foods they come into contact with, especially when heated. Most foods you pick up in grocery stores and delis, such as meats, cheeses and sandwiches, are wrapped in PVC.

Consider that cling wrap is made of PVC plastic. The leftover meatloaf you eat that was wrapped in this plastic may now contain toxic chemicals that have been found to cause reproductive problems, birth defects, liver tumors and hormonal disruptions in mice. This is especially true if you reheat the meatloaf in the plastic wrap in a microwave oven. The longer the meatloaf sits in the plastic, the more toxins leach into it, and the more toxins you eat when you have your meatloaf sandwich a few days later. Although more research into this issue is justified, it doesn't seem to be a high priority with the FDA at this time.

From a prevention standpoint, there seems to be enough concern and evidence to suggest that plastics can and do contribute to toxins in our food, in our bodies, and in our environment. This is reason enough for me to encourage folks to be careful about how they store and reheat their food, and what kinds of containers they buy their food in (because grocery store foods can sit in warehouses, on shipping vehicles and on store shelves for long periods of time). Glass storage containers with lids are an excellent and safe alternative for storing, reheating and freezing foods. They are dishwasher safe, reusable, and transportable. When buying "to go" or freezer foods in a store, select those that are stored in cardboard and in such a way that the food is not in direct contact with the plastic outer wrapping, if they have one. Avoid using Styrofoam cups and plates (especially with hot foods and beverages, even though they are marketed for this purpose), and plastic plates and utensils. For picnics, choose paper plates and consider using your own kitchen cutlery or wooden utensils instead of plastic.

Several years ago, *The Green Guide*, a newsletter with information about toxic-free living, came out with a comprehensive list of which plastic products to choose and avoid. If you look on the bottom of plastic food storage containers, you will see a number and/or some letters. That code tells you what kind of plastic the container is made of. In general, for water and food storage, look for plastics that are labeled as #1 (PETE), #2 (HDPE), #4 (LDPE), or #5 (PP) and avoid those labeled as #3 (PVC), #6 (PS), and #7 (Polycarbonate). You can visit www.mothers.org and www.checnet.org (the Children's Health Environment Coalition) for more information on topics such as this.

Concluding Comments on Nutrition

Overall, researchers who have studied the connection between nutrition and children's behavior have found that dietary and nutritional changes help many, but not all of the subjects. My belief is that any changes in diet or nutrition need to be based on each person's unique body chemistry, history, etc., with specific treatments geared toward their individual needs. Trying to pick one diet, vitamin, mineral, or other supplement to give to everyone with similar symptoms is not, in my opinion, safe or smart. The uniqueness of each person, and the fact that similar symptoms can be linked to very different things for different people, makes this "one treatment fits all" practice seem careless and irresponsible. That is why it is so important to work with a naturopath, holistic doctor, clinical nutritionist or other health professional that can assess your child's profile of symptoms and choose the treatments that will be most aligned with their special needs.

In my view, the success that professionals and the research are showing with diet and nutritional changes in optimizing children's development is too great to ignore. I imagine that (rather than being an indication that diet and nutrition are not factors in the symptoms of such diagnoses as AD/HD) some of the variance in this area of research is due to people's individual differences, and to the fact that we try to put a group of very unique people into one category. It seems to me that when you bring your brain and body functions into balance with a personal nutritional program, you are getting to what might be at the "root" of the problem, rather than simply using drugs to calm symptoms for a short period of time. Since it is a safe, natural, and gentle choice, it seems a good early start to looking for solutions to addressing issues such as those linked to the AD/HD diagnosis.

7

RELAXATION AND EXERCISE

Using them to balance children's wellbeing

SCIENTISTS TODAY HAVE proven that a strong connection exists between the state of our mental health and the state of our physical health. We generally call this the "mind-body connection." What we think, so we become. Our thoughts, emotions, physical and spiritual wellbeing are linked as an inseparable whole. Our mental, emotional, physical, spiritual, and energetic bodies are in constant communication with each other, responding to each other's signals.

This same principal goes for our life experiences in general. If you spend your day thinking negative thoughts, your day will likely be filled with negative experiences, and if you spend your day thinking positive thoughts, your day will likely be filled with positive experiences. Scientists and quantum physicists call this general principle "the Law of Attraction."

The Law of Attraction is what we call a "Universal Law" – like gravity. You can't see it, but you know it exists and you know it works. The Law of Attraction basically says that "like attracts like." Positive energy sent out to the Universe in the form of thoughts, words or deeds attracts more positive energy, and the same for the negative – not because they are either positive or negative, but because the Universe only "sees" the energy patterns of these things, not their form (i.e., positive or negative), and then sends you more of it. The Law of Attraction says that whatever energy pattern the Universe sees you expressing is exactly what you'll get more of. It's an unfailing law, according to quantum physicists.

So when thinking about you and your child's health, this simple concept can be very powerful. Whatever "vibes" you send into the Universe will create more of that same "vibe." When you and your child are stressed, and all of your energies are going into being or feeling stressed, the Universe thinks that's what you want more of, so that's what you get. You don't *really* want more stress in your child's life, so how can you shift this? Let's take a look at ways to bring this part of your child's health into balance again.

Relaxation

Today, everybody knows the importance of making time for relaxation. Whether we are young or old, the time we take to rest is part of what keeps us in a vibrant state of health. Relaxation time lets all the parts of ourselves rebuild and get strong so that we can keep doing everything we choose to do in a healthy way. Our bodies intuitively know that rest is a necessary part of their ability to function properly. Dr. Herbert Benson, a cardiologist at Harvard University, calls the body's natural tendency to unwind when at rest the "relaxation response."

Remember that we are made up of five "bodies" that form our whole selves: the physical, the mental or psychological, the emotional, the spiritual, and the energetic. Stress can show up in any or all of these bodies as physical exhaustion, mental overwhelm, emotional distress, spiritual conflict or behavioral "outbursts," for example. When we are stressed and we do not make time for relaxation, we wear ourselves out. In fact, on the physical level, stress contributes to ulcers, heart disease, insomnia, high blood pressure, and back and chest pain in the body. There is also evidence that chronic stress can weaken the immune system. Stress in the mental body can show up as confusion, overwhelm, inability to make decisions, forgetfulness, distractibility, disorientation, or mental meandering. When the emotional body is stressed, a person might experience anxiety, restlessness, discomfort or uneasiness, moodiness, withdrawal, panic, a sense of urgency, anger, sadness or weepiness, dissociation, or detachment from themselves or others.

Stress in the spiritual/energetic realm typically results from an inner conflict between one or more of the "ruling" parts of the psyche and what we call the Higher Self (our Divine Soul, Spirit or Life Force; that sacred spark of life within us). To borrow Freudian terms, the "ruling" parts of our psyche include the id (our unconscious thoughts and beliefs), the ego (our conscious thoughts and beliefs), and the superego (our internal "judge"). This inner conflict creates energy in our bodies that must be released. Generally, energy born of inner conflict or distress is released through behaviors that are inappropriate, "toxic," or unhealthy for ourselves or others.

When we are overly stressed, we begin to lose our sense of who we are and what we are about. We begin to question what we are doing in the world. We become uncomfortable with our life choices or situation, yet are not certain how to change it. We become aware that what we truly want and feel for ourselves inside is not consistent with the life we are living. This is when our stress has reached a spiritual level – the most intense and meaningful for most of us. Some general signs of stress are listed below.

Our bodies are set up to work in perfect harmony and to self-correct when something is wrong. The relaxation response is just one example of this self-healing directive. When we are overly stressed, the body will give us warning signals to let us know that we are about to have a "meltdown," or lapse of health in our state of being. If we ignore these signals (for example, headaches, stomachaches, illnesses, accidents, lack of energy, appetite or sleep changes, chronic fatigue, moodiness, random aches and pains, drug/alcohol [ab]use), we may find ourselves in a crisis shortly thereafter. If we do not take notice and make changes in our lifestyle, not only do we end up suffering, but so do the people and things that are most important to us. We may even lose them completely.

General Signs of Dis-stress

Physical	Stiff, sore muscles; Muscle tension; Muscle fatigue; Headaches; Quick or shallow breathing; Pounding or rapid heart beat; Overeating; Loss of appetite; Sleep difficulties; Digestion problems; Physical exhaustion; Lethargy; Low productivity; Increased accidents; Always in motion or rushing; Restlessness; Anxiety; Nervous tension; Fidgety, twitchy; Inability to relax
Mental	Difficulty concentrating; Wondering mind; Distractibility; "Spacing out" or daydreaming; Forgetfulness; Apathy; Boredom; Dulled senses; "Dumb" mistakes; Difficulty making decisions; Confusion; Negativity; Pessimism; Focus on what's not OK rather than what is OK; Mental exhaustion; Lack of motivation
Emotional	Frustration; Irritability; "Short fuse"; Lashing out; Fussiness; Anger; Nagging; Moody; Intolerant; Resentful; Emotional exhaustion; Overwhelm; Anxiety; Easily discouraged; Depression; The "blues"; Crying spells; Flat affect; Negativity; Lack of joy; Easily discouraged
Behavioral	Apathy; Loss of sense of self; Social isolation; Increased use of substances; Negative self-Talk; Self-doubt; Feeling shame; Feeling guilt; Feeling worthless; Lack of meaning; Lack of purpose; Conflicting ideas; Conflicting needs; Fear; Anger; Anxiety; Sense of stagnation; Sense of longing; Sense of emptiness; Loss of sense of security; Loss of sense of stability; Feeling "lost"; Feeling hopeless; Feeling alone; Lashing out; Isolating; Avoiding; Aggressing; Unpredictable; Unreliable; Lack of Presence

Children and adolescents have fewer coping skills than most adults to deal with life when they are stressed. They tend to show their discomfort through their behavior and their moods. For example, they may get ornery, angry, and rebellious. They may "push your buttons." They may argue or throw tantrums. Their sleeping and eating patterns might change. They may not listen or do what they are told. They may forget things. They may be disorganized. They can become irrational. They might isolate themselves or be gone all the time. They will likely complain, blame, and become negative about everything. Any request feels like too much for them to do, so they often create a reason not to do it at all; they create a distraction. Aggression and/or violent behavior toward others might increase. This type of behavior can be symptomatic of any number of diagnosable disorders, including what we call AD/HD.

Just as with adults, if chronic, intense stress is not addressed with a youngster, they will eventually suffer a lapse or relapse in some area of their lives. The stress-energy they are trying to contain in their body will have to be discharged somewhere, some how, some time. They may fail school or lose a job. They might become verbally or physically abusive to themselves or others. They might lose an important relationship. They might get physically ill. They could get in trouble with the law or go to jail. They could disappear or run away in search of relief. They might begin to abuse drugs or alcohol, or engage in other risky behaviors. Basically, just as with adults, they could "lose it" or explode one day and cause pain to themselves or others. Sometimes, the damage created as a result of such an outburst cannot be repaired. That is why it is *so* important for parents and caregivers to be aware of the signs of distress in youngsters so that they can get help and begin to heal before a crisis occurs.

Being a child in today's world is very demanding. Each year, schools raise their expectations, families get busier and spend a lot of time apart, and there are new dangers to deal with. Getting a "good night's sleep" is difficult for many children, due to family stress, unsafe neighborhoods, issues related to poverty, abuse and neglect factors, or simply "busy-ness." The speed of everything seems to be increasing. It takes a lot of energy to keep up.

Just like adults, children have an easier time doing their best each day when they take time to relax, unwind, and "de-stress." It is chronic (day after day), severe stress that feels the worst, but even small amounts of stress over time can create problems. Situational stress that is born out of an acute (one time) traumatic event, such as the death of a loved one, divorce, a move, loss of a loved pet, changing schools or neighborhoods, an accident, or abuse, can also be devastating.

Symptoms resulting from situational stress are easier to identify, since they can be linked to a specific event. In cases where the symptoms of situational stress or trauma do not show signs of decreasing within six months after the event, other emotional or spiritual/behavioral issues may have developed that require attention (such as symptoms of an *Adjustment Disorder* or *Major Depressive Episode*). For these reasons, it is very important to provide youngsters with a safe place to "vent" or release their stress energy on a regular basis. From a holistic health care model, this type of prevention is the first line of intervention.

Working to contain "stress energy" saps the body's healthy energy reserves that are used for functioning and self-healing. On the other hand, releasing stress energy in a safe way frees a person from having to work at containing it within their body. This is why making time for stress release and relaxation is so important. Scheduling regular time for renewal will give the body an opportunity to use its relaxation response. This can prevent the development of stress-related symptoms.

If every day is not possible, then fit in some time whenever it *is* possible. Even if you can only find 15 minutes once a week, it will make a positive difference. One time a week is better than no time. If you can keep this up for a few weeks, you will begin to wonder how you ever lived without it in the first place. You and your child will likely begin to look forward to that special time, and choose to extend or increase it. Making time for the self is one way to show that you honor and respect yourself, which is a great role model for children. To honor and respect the self allows us to honor and respect others. Then, we can begin to live more compassionate, peaceful, and loving lives.

A good place to start with your child is to ask them to name some things they find relaxing and talk to them about their choices. You could also ask them about things that are stressful to them and talk about ideas for taking the stress away. You can model healthy ways to relax, and encourage your child to find some that work for them. Pick a few that are safe, easy to do, and easy to work into your days. Then find a slot of time to schedule them in for a few weeks. This is a powerful life skill for you and your child to practice. Taking time for the self to renew and revive is very empowering on many levels of being. In this chapter, you will find examples of things to consider and others to avoid. Try some for a week or two and feel the difference!

Preventing Stress

"Prevention is the best intervention." This is my motto for stress management. There are so many small life changes that you and your child can make to keep yourselves healthy and happy, while preventing the build-up of unhealthy stress. Keep in mind that a certain amount of "stress" is actually healthy. It keeps us from feeling bored, depressed, tired, or "numb" to life around us. It is only when we get *too much* stress in our lives that it becomes unhealthy. With a healthy amount of stress, we are happy, creative, motivated, productive, and physically sound. Here are some easy ways to prevent the development of unhealthy stress in your child's life and make it easier for them be their best:

1. **Get enough rest:** Try to give children between 6 and 8 hours of sleep each night. Have them take a nap on their days off to let their body catch up on missed sleep. Remember: sufficient sleep is necessary for healthy living; it is not an option. It allows the body time to rejuvenate, and stay strong and healthy.

2. **Eat healthy:** Reduce or eliminate the influences of tobacco, caffeine, alcohol, sugar, and salt; they increase body stress. Add in more organic fruits, vegetables, nuts, whole grains, beans, and dairy foods.

3.   **Exercise regularly:** At least 20 minutes 3 days a week is best to get the heart pumping and the body moving (e.g., walking, riding a bike, climbing stairs, jumping jacks, basketball, jumping rope, skipping).

4.   **Take time to relax:** Teach children to use a relaxation technique regularly (e.g., positive self-talk, counting, deep breathing, meditation, visualization, pleasant imagery, progressive muscle relaxation, yoga; read on for more examples).

5.   **Adjust your attitude:** Teach children to think positively, for instance, make a point to "see the glass full or half full" rather than "empty or half empty."

6.   **Pamper them:** Take time to do something special just for your child so they can "refill" (e.g., take a bath, eat something yummy, write a letter, call a friend, buy something new, go somewhere special).

7.   **Affirm them:** For example, tell them, "You are enough; you have enough; you do enough" every day.

8.   **Be kind to them:** Humans cannot achieve perfection, nor do we need to; we can strive to be our best at any given moment, and know that it is enough. Go easy on your children. They are doing their best. Support them in using "mistakes" to learn, grow and expand from. Teach kids to live, forgive, learn, and love themselves.

Ways to Relax And Rebuild

Relaxation is very important for children. To them, the world can be a stressful place with many demands to handle every day. It is important to teach children how to create "down time" in their lives, as a way of managing stress. Down time cannot be rushed, and it works best when it is not attached to a task of any kind. If it is, it becomes just another stressor. Basically, the art of relaxing involves taking time to do something positive that is *only* for you and your well being… not for anyone or anything else. It means creating a window of time that is devoted to the self, because you are worth it, whether you are five or fifty years old.

Relaxation can be many things. Although it can involve naps, rest time, or quiet time (with no audio or visual stimuli like TV, music, or computers), it does not have to mean that kids must lie down and take "quiet time." Sometimes moving, stretching, and bending the body is the best way to relax it. Relaxation can mean taking a leisurely walk or a bike ride. It could be dancing, paying for a professional massage, or joining a special group or team that meets regularly. It might be a bubble bath, reading a special book or magazine, listening to calm music, gardening, or watching the critters in your yard. It might be meditating or sitting quietly in front of a candle, doing yoga or Qigong, writing in a journal, drawing, or simply working on a creative project that has special meaning, with no time limits for getting it done.

There are so many ways to relax – about as many ways as there are people in the world. I have included a few "tried and true" methods in this section that I use with the school-aged children I work with. Even the most active children are wonderful at meditating and doing mental visualizations. Some, but not all of the ideas I have included, can be used with preschoolers. You are the expert on your child. You know better than anyone what types of activities will work with them and what types won't. Use your judgment and be willing to experiment. I trust that you will find something that works for you and your child. If you want to learn more about relaxation methods for children, check your local bookstore. There are wonderful books, audio and video tapes for teaching children meditation, yoga, and other relaxation methods.

Micro-breaks: Here is a list of twenty ways to help your child (and yourself) relax that can be done for a minute or less and still make a positive difference in how they feel. I call them "micro-breaks":

1. Look out of a window. Mentally review the details of what you see.
2. Step out into the sun and sit down or take a mini-walk.
3. Make "angel-wings" with your arms.
4. Shake out your legs or kick them up and down.

5. Massage tight muscles.
6. Rest your eyes (rub your hands together briskly to warm your palms; then, hold your palms over closed eyes).
7. Hum, sing or whistle a few bars of a favorite song.
8. Close your eyes, put your head down, and be silent.
9. Breathe deeply (use abdominal breathing).
10. Play with a small, manipulative toy (e.g., squishy ball, bubbles, slinky).
11. Have a healthy snack (anything without sugar, caffeine, or salt, such as unsalted nuts, fruit, carrots, cheese and crackers, unsalted popcorn).
12. Lightly "stimulate" your head, neck or face with your hands or fingertips (this means softly "slapping" or tapping your head, neck and face, rather than rubbing).
13. Spritz or splash your face with plain water or water scented with a favorite stimulating or relaxing essential oil.
14. Say positive or affirming things to yourself (e.g., "I am a productive worker," "I get things done," or "I am a good person.")
15. Put a smile on your face for no reason except that it will make you feel better.
16. Light a candle (with a favorite relaxing or stimulating scent):
    Relaxing: Chamomile, Lavender, Rose, Sage, Sandalwood, Orange Blossom
    Stimulating: Peppermint, Lemon, Spearmint, Eucalyptus, Jasmine, Geranium
17. Lie down and stretch your arms over your head. Rest your body, mind, emotions, and spirit.
18. Laugh or chuckle out loud just because you can.
19. Think of something kind that you can do or say to someone else today.
20. Think of something that you can be thankful for today.

Relaxation Using The Breath

There are many simple ways to get your child to relax that do not take much effort on their part. One way is by using the breath. Many relaxation techniques involve breathing more naturally, from the abdomen. This way of breathing can be used to relax during times of stress or anxiety. Here, I describe a few breathing exercises for relaxation that are fairly easy for children to learn and apply.

Deep Breathing: Children can begin to relax by taking some time to learn a different way of breathing. Most of our breathing is very shallow - held up in the lungs. When the average person takes a breath, their lungs expand and contract with the air before their diaphragm and abdomen. This way of breathing, however, is unnatural and inefficient. The healthier and more natural way to breathe is called, "diaphragmatic or abdominal" breathing. This method of deep breathing means that the air is pulled in and pushed out under the leadership of the diaphragm and the abdomen, rather than the lungs. The diaphragm and the abdomen expand with each inhale to make space for the fresh air to come in, and contract with each exhale to push out the stale air held in our bodies (followed by the lungs).

Natural, deep breathing is physically more efficient and nurturing for our bodies. According to Ravi Singh, a leading Kundalini Yoga instructor in the U.S., long, deep breathing fuels our metabolism, feeds our blood, helps to clear out impurities from our bodies, is a tonic for our nervous system, helps balance the pH levels of our blood, and massages our inner organs. Singh also argues that it releases emotional blocks that may be held in our muscles, and helps keep the spine aligned through the creation of "micro-movements" (small, subtle movements in the spinal structure). Children can learn natural breathing by practicing the following exercise:

> **Exercise:** To breathe more naturally, you want to pull the air down into your belly when you inhale, and release the air from your belly when you exhale. When you breath in this way, your belly should expand and fill with air before your lungs do on the inhale, and contract and empty of air before your lungs do on the exhale. Belly breathing means that your breath is lead by the belly rather than the lungs. While you are

learning this breath, it helps to consciously expand your belly on the in-hale and contract it on the exhale. With practice, it will not take you long to begin breathing this way automatically.

Once your child masters the art of natural, abdominal (or belly) breathing, there are many ways to enhance the positive effects of the breath for their physical, mental, emotional, spiritual, and energetic wellbeing. Here are a few suggestions:

Eight Breathing Exercises for Relaxation
Close your eyes and find a quiet place to do your breathing.

1. Take at least three long, deep abdominal breaths.

2. Hold each inhale to the count of three (1-1000, 2-1000, 3-1000) before exhaling.

3. Inhale to the count of six, and exhale to the count of six to slow your breathing down. Build up to a count of twelve if you wish.

4. Inhale to the count of six, hold your breath to the count of three, and exhale to the count of six. Build up to the count of twelve if you wish.

5. Think positive thoughts while you breathe (e.g., "I did a lot today.").

6. Imagine a pleasant scene or recall a pleasant memory while you breathe.

7. Think positive affirmations while you breathe (e.g., "I am healthy.").

8. "Shift" your throat when you inhale and exhale to a place somewhere between a normal breath and a snore. When you breathe normally, there is usually little or no sound. When you snore, there is a lot of sound. In between these two places, we can "shift" our throats to breathe with a soft sound that is comparable to a "half-snore." It should be a whispery or breathy sound rather than a snoring sound. Doing this will help to pull the air down deep into your abdomen. This is the most relaxing type of breathing.

There is an excellent little book by breath and movement expert Lauren Robins, titled *The Palette of Breath: Facts About Breathing*. Ms. Robins has a Master's degree in Education, is a massage therapist, and teaches yoga, dance, movement, and breath classes to all ages. Her book is filled with healthy facts about what she calls "belly breathing," or abdominal breathing. It is written in a fun way that appeals to children and is easy to understand. In the book, Ms. Robins links the breath with opening up all parts of ourselves, including our mental, emotional, physical, spiritual, and energetic bodies. It provides an easy way for parents to teach children about being self-aware and self-nurturing, and it is also a nice introduction for going deeper with the breathing exercises described in this chapter.

Relaxation Using The Mind

There are many relaxation techniques available for children who can be still and use their minds in a creative way. I review several choices here that work well with children and are easy to learn.

Counting: Counting is a very simple way for children to calm down quickly, and it is scientifically proven to be effective. The process is easy: count forward from zero to twenty ("Forward Counting"), or backward from twenty to zero ("Backward Counting"), either silently or aloud (e.g., "1-1000, 2-1000,… 20-1000," or "20-1000, 19-1000,… 1-1000"). Each count should take about one second's time. It may not be as effective if your child rushes through it, so encourage them to go slowly, which is why you add the "1000" to the count. If they are so upset or stressed that they resist this simple exercise, I suggest they take a few deep breaths, too.

Positive Self-Talk: This is the art of "seeing the glass full or half-full" rather than "empty or half-empty." There are two parts to this relaxation technique that children can learn: 1) stop thinking and saying negative things, and 2) replace their negative thoughts and words with positive ones. For instance, if your child is stressed about something they must do, help them stop and "listen" to the messages they may be telling themselves. Check for negative self-talk (e.g., "I can't do this! This scares me. I am not ready for this. How can I get this done on time?"). Next, help them replace those thoughts with positive ones (e.g., "O.K. Calm down. I can do this! I have confidence in myself. I am ready for this. I will find a way to get this done on time."). You get the idea. This can be helpful in any number of situations. Once their attitude shifts into something more positive and calming, their physical and emotional states should relax, too.

Transcendental Meditation®: Transcendental Meditation® is one form of meditation that has been shown in the research to help with many of the symptoms linked to the AD/HD diagnosis. Specifically, it can support the body by improving brain and mental functioning, calming the nervous system and decreasing stress. Research also shows that it supports more positive feelings about the self and others, decreases nervousness, and may discourage drug and alcohol use. It does this by teaching a natural state of restful-alertness to the person doing the meditation, and helps them to stay calm and focused in the midst of activity. Anyone age 10 or older can learn this type of meditation, which is usually practiced twice a day for 10 to 20 minutes. Consult your bookstore for more information about this particular method.

Meditation: Transcendental Meditation® is not the only type that can help with relaxation, rejuvenation and focus. There are a number of yoga meditations and other visualization techniques that can be used, too. Check your local bookstore for resources on meditation, including books, and audio and videotapes. One of my favorites is *Earthlight, New Meditations for Children,* by Maureen Garth, who wrote this special book for parents to teach their children how to meditate. She also taught, wrote books about meditation for teenagers and adults, and was a speaker on the subject of meditation for many years until her death in 1997. Here is a sample from part of the opening meditation in *Earthlight*:

The Star Prelude:

I want you to see above your head a beautiful, beautiful Star. This star is very special to you, as it is your very own Star. It can be any color ... or colors you choose. This special Star is filled with white light, lovely white light which shimmers and glows. I want you to see this light streaming down toward you until it reaches the very top of your head. And now I want you to bring this pure light down through your head and take it right down your body until your whole body is filled with this glorious white light...

This meditation goes on to introduce children to their Guardian Angel, who takes them with safety past the Worry Tree (who takes all of their worries for them) and into their very own garden, where anything enjoyable can be done. Although the meditations in this book are sweet, beautiful, and enjoyable for children, they can really be used with any age.

The following is a very simple way of teaching your child to achieve a state of relaxation through a different kind of meditation:

Exercise: Sit or lie down comfortably in a quiet place and breathe long and deeply (abdominally). Slow down your breathing so that each inhale and exhale lasts to the count of six (1-1000, 2-1000, 3-1000...). For extra relaxation, you can hold to the count of three between the inhale and exhale. Take at least three breaths this way, before beginning a rhythmic long, deep breathing pattern at your own pace. Focus your mind on something peaceful or relaxing. It could be a prayer, a saying, an affirmation, or a song. It could be the image of a spiritual role model. Think about what the words, sounds, or symbols mean to you. Think about how to apply the messages or teachings they hold for you in your own life. Continue for at least 15 minutes with closed eyes.

To "come out" of meditation from a sitting position, inhale while slowly stretching your arms up over your head. Hold the breath and this position until you are ready to exhale. Then, slowly lower your arms with the exhale. Open your eyes, sit quietly for a minute, and resume a natural breath. To come out of a meditation from a lying down position, inhale and stretch your arms up over your head, and your legs out with pointed toes. Hold this position until you are ready to exhale. Then, relax your arms to your sides and your legs to the ground. Bring your knees up to your chest and hold your shins with your hands. Then, slowly rock yourself up to a sitting position. Or, bend your knees with your feet flat on the ground, roll over to one side and gently push yourself up with your arms.

Progressive Muscle Relaxation: This form of meditation is a popular and easy way to relax the muscles in the body. I have found that it works well with young children and teenagers who are "wound up." I suggest doing this exercise with your child at first, so that you can do it with them and be their model:

Exercise: Have your child sit or lie down in a comfortable, quiet place and close their eyes. You can start with any muscle group in the body, but I recommend beginning at the top and working your way down to the feet. For example, focus your attention on your head and facial muscles. Inhale and tense the muscles as much as possible. This means making silly faces! Hold the tension for 5 seconds. Then release the tension with the exhale to a count of 5, and let the muscles relax. Repeat this two more times before moving down to the neck muscles. Continue with each muscle group, finishing with the toes and feet, until your body feels completely relaxed.

Revisit any area that is still holding tension after you have gone over your entire body once. Lightly massage the area and repeat the exercise for that particular body part. In your mind, "talk" to the tense body part. Thank it for getting your attention, and tell it that it is O.K. to let go and relax now. This may sound silly, but in doing so, you send a message from your brain to the cells, muscles, and related tissue of the body part to help it relax and return to a more natural state of functioning.

Visualization: Visualization is a type of meditation that uses the "mind's eye" to take you on a mental journey. As with meditation, there are books and audiotapes you can buy at your local bookstore to guide you through different kinds of visualizations. Like Progressive Muscle Relaxation, I have had good results from using this with children and adolescents. Here is a simple visualization that can be combined with Progressive Muscle Relaxation if you'd like. This one can easily be done in a small family group:

Exercise: Sit or lie down in a comfortable, quiet place and close your eyes. Take three long, deep breaths. See in your mind's eye your abdomen and your lungs filling with air as you breathe -- filling and emptying -- in a smooth, flowing rhythm. Continue to focus on your breath. Envision the muscles of your head, face, and neck holding knots and tension. Then, picture the knots and the tension releasing with each exhale. In your mind's eye, watch the knots and tension exit your body with your breath. Breathe in relaxing, renewing energy; breathe out the muscle tension. One at a time, envision this process with each part of your body, beginning with your head and moving down to your feet and toes. Continue for at least 10 minutes.

Pleasant Imagery: Like Visualization, this technique is also a type of meditation. It is used in certain types of therapy for reducing anxiety and stress. Although similar to the Visualization technique, it has a slightly different purpose. With Pleasant Imagery, the focus is on literally taking a mental journey to a place or experience that brings children a sense of joy and peace. It can be imaginary or an actual place or experience they had. The purpose is to give their brain and body a break from the stress in their life and take them to a place where they can re-experience a positive state of being:

Exercise: Find a quiet place to sit or lie down, and close your eyes. Focus your thoughts on either something that you remember or something that you imagine as being a very comfortable and pleasant experience for you. Think of all the details that you can about the situation. Let your thoughts lead you to actual images in your mind about what it is like. Notice the sounds, smells, colors, tastes, or other sensations that you experience in the situation. Try to imagine yourself in that place or situation. Hold on to the fantasy and the pleasant feelings that you experience there for at least five minutes and let your body relax into them.

Relaxation Through Movement

If you feel that something involving movement will work best for your child, yoga and Qigong are two good choices to consider. They combine meditation with breathing and movement to provide whole-body relaxation and revitalization. Here, I provide a brief review of each of these relaxation techniques.

Yoga: There are many types of yoga, and many levels to choose from. Anyone from children to elders, from beginner to advanced, can find a yoga class, tape or book on the market today that will match their needs. Yoga combines physical, mental, emotional, spiritual, and energetic elements to empower and strengthen the self. Some types, such as Hatha Yoga, focus on stretching and postures to stimulate the organs, strengthen the muscles, stretch the tendons and ligaments, nourish the central nervous system, and clear the lymphatic system. Others, such as Kundalini Yoga, focus on specialized breathing along with postures, to stimulate different energy centers and organs, oxygenate the blood, clear the lungs, help the body detoxify, and put the systems of your body in sync. Kundalini Yoga also emphasizes connection to the "Higher Power", or God, within and outside of the self. Most types are intended to help the systems of the body remain in a general state of balance and harmony. Many types also involve meditation or prayer (silently or aloud), which may include chanting, toning, or singing.

As a regular practitioner of Hatha and Kundalini Yoga since 2000, I can vouch for the positive life changes it can bring about. For me, these have included physical strength and stamina, flexibility, mental clarity, emotional calm and stability (even during times of high stress), inner peace, a stronger sense of self, confidence, a more positive attitude and outlook, and more loving feelings about the self, others, and the world. My belief is that only when we can truly connect with, love, respect, forgive, nurture, and be compassionate toward ourselves, can we extend these gifts to those outside of ourselves (e.g., people, animals, the environment, our community, and the world around us). The practice of yoga is one healthy way to begin this very personal journey.

Qigong: Although the practice of Qigong (pronounced "Chi-gong") came to the US during the past 20 years, it is a form of movement, breathing and meditation that has been used for the prevention and treatment of illness and disease in China since at least c.600 B.C. Dr. Tom Williams says in his book, *The Complete Illustrated Guide to Chinese Medicine*, that to the Chinese, "Qi" is "the vital life energy responsible for healthy functioning of the body...(it) is everywhere all the time: flowing, permeating, and energizing everything in the universe, including our bodies." Qigong, then, is a method of increasing the "efficiency and effectiveness of how we store, move, and use Qi to enhance our health and wellbeing."[5]

Since Qigong was preserved and passed down through the ruling families and the Daoist and Buddhist monasteries in China, the thousands of forms have been expanded and modified, yet they all share a common purpose:

- rebuilding Qi;
- balancing Qi, to clear blocks or excesses; and
- reinforcing internal and external Qi (internally, making sure the systems of the body are flowing smoothly; externally, building up Qi energy to protect the body).
- Overall, the exercises promote health and longevity in people of all ages. As with other Chinese systems of movement (such as T'ai Chi), Qigong has been proven as an effective way to prevent and cure illness in the body.

Some of the forms are short, and for this reason, may work better with children than say, T'ai Chi or even Karate. Qigong exercises can be learned from a good book or video, but a teacher can be a better way to go, especially for children. Here are a few things to consider when choosing a teacher. Find one who:

1. has been teaching children for at least three years;
2. understands and follows the principles of Chinese philosophy;
3. can provide individual attention and teaching to your child;
4. you are comfortable with;
5. and whose mission is clear.

Activities to Avoid

There are certain activities that I suggest parents avoid when selecting a relaxation technique. That is because true relaxation activities cannot be attached to something else that needs to be done. Although this might seem efficient to the busy parent, it does not generally work for the child. I mention a few common activities that parents are tempted to use here:

Task-Oriented Projects: Avoid making household chores or tasks into relaxation activities. For example, not everyone would find raking the leaves or weeding the garden relaxing. Make sure your child is allowed to pick activities that are relaxing to *them*, and not attached to another task that needs to be done. Whatever they choose, make sure they will have enough time to do it, are prepared to end when it's time, or that they are comfortable continuing it another day. You do not want them to feel disturbed or rushed through their relaxation activity. That would defeat the purpose altogether.

Shopping and other costly activities: Although shopping excursions with the kids may be fun sometimes, it is usually not relaxing. Avoid using shopping, or any other activity that involves money (e.g., movies, skating, eating out, arcades), for a relaxation activity. This can get costly and may be stressful, tiring, or over-stimulating instead of relaxing. Kids who are used to high amounts of stimulation (for example, from television, videos, or computer games) may require extra guidance and coaching when selecting activities they would like to do for relaxation. It may feel strange for them to engage in something that is calm and quiet instead of "fast and furious." For those individuals who are not used to it, the art of relaxing must be learned, just as any new skill does.

Multi-child activities: Doing relaxing things as a family or inviting friends along may save time and energy, but it may not be productive. It is too difficult to please everyone, and compromising can become stressful. Even if you play a favorite family game, if it is a competitive game, someone will end up losing, which may leave them feeing more stressed. Unless you reserve "quiet time" or a "quiet hour" at your house, in which everyone observes silence, multi-person activities do not work well for relaxation. Let each person pick their own time and their own activity whenever possible. This may mean that everyone agrees to honor and respect each other's relaxation time. The key is for relaxation time to be individual, special, self-rewarding, *and* relaxing.

Punishment: However tempting it may be, do not attach relaxation time to a punishment. For instance, parents may be tempted to make a child's "Time Out" or "Time Away" their relaxation time. Grounding a child to their room, or telling them to go lay down on their bed and calm down, are also not what I mean by relaxation time. There is a huge difference between doing something especially chosen for relaxation and doing something as part of a punishment. Do not mix the two.

Final Thoughts About Relaxation

Science has shown us what a health hazard stress is. Stressful living is responsible for many people's illnesses and health problems. Taking the time to relax is a powerful prevention tool. Like adults, children's lives – school – can feel stressful to them. School is a very demanding place on many levels for children. It takes a great deal of courage to get through a school day. Children may be asked to do things that challenge, scare, or embarrass them. They deal with crowds of people each day, not all of them friendly. They constantly get feedback about whether they are "right" or "wrong," "successful" or "unsuccessful," "appropriate" or "inappropriate." They may worry about appearing foolish or stupid to their classmates and teachers. They must keep up with their work, supplies and their schedule. Even children who enjoy school and find it "easy" must maneuver their way through a number of tricky situations each day.

Children can benefit from relaxation as much as adults can. Children can learn the important skill of how to balance the busyness in their lives with relaxation. Their bodies, like our bodies, need a certain amount of time to unwind, rest, and rebuild. Sleep provides some of this, but sometimes sleep alone is not enough. Relaxation time can support kids in being and doing their best each day. Helping children understand the value of making and taking the time to relax is something that they can benefit from their entire lives.

Exercise

We have all heard about the benefits of regular exercise for our well-being. Most health professionals include exercise in their list of preventatives for any number of health issues. The benefits of exercise have been consistently proven with scientific research. There is no longer any question about the body's need for some type of regular physical activity to keep it healthy and strong. This is especially important for growing bodies, and is a healthy way for active youngsters to "burn off some steam." When the body is healthy and properly oxygenated, it does its best and allows us to do our best. A healthy body is less likely to show signs of stress, such as those that are related to the symptoms of an AD/HD diagnosis.

Stephen C. Putnam, who has a Master of Education degree in Guidance and Psychological Services, is an advocate of exercise for health and fun. In his book, *Nature's Ritalin for the Marathon Mind: Nurturing your ADHD Child with Exercise*, he writes that children who respond well to psycho-stimulants also generally respond well to exercise. As with other options, exercise alone will not get rid of AD/HD-like symptoms. There is strong evidence, however, that it is a vital part of brain functioning and health, which is an essential element of addressing children's symptoms. I refer you to his book for a detailed look at the role of exercise in treating symptoms related to the AD/HD diagnosis.

There are many reasons why we are more sedentary as a people than ever before. Putnam reviews these in his book, and questions whether it is simply coincidence that as life has gotten "easier" and our need for routine exercise has greatly decreased, our society has become more and more reliant on chemicals. Could there be a correlation between movement and mental health? Absolutely. We *know* that exercise affects the level and functioning of neurotransmitters in the brain; it affects neurochemistry. It does the same thing that pharmaceutical drugs do; it increases the amount of certain neurotransmitters in the brain.

Does this mean that exercise is the answer to your child's AD/HD-like symptoms? Not necessarily. Exercise, although beneficial for everyone, has a unique impact based on each person's situation. The degree to which it may help your child is dependant on many personal and environmental factors in your child's life. Unless your child's doctor specifically warns against participation in physical exercise for a medical reason, exercise cannot harm them, and *will* help them to some degree. Regular exercise may calm their energy, elevate their mood, improve their ability to focus, increase their motivation, and give them some fun. It can be a very positive part of not only your child's life, but of your own.

Benefits of Exercise

On a mental-emotional level, research shows that regular exercise helps relieve anxiety, depression, and stress. It can improve self-esteem and elevate mood. It makes us feel good: exercise "increases blood flow to the brain, releases hormones, stimulates the nervous system, and increases levels of morphine-like substances found in the body...that can have a positive effect on mood and create a neurophysiological high,"[6] according to Michael H. Sacks, M.D. We feel more in control, confident, and effective. It strengthens our ability to deal with emotional stress. Just knowing that we have done something positive and nurturing for ourselves during a busy day of doing for others, can lift our spirits. It works the same way for children.

On a physical and energetic level, exercise can improve overall physical fitness and resilience, improve or protect the functioning of the body's immune system, improve heart and lung capacity, and decrease muscle tension. The right amount of exercise can have a relaxing or tranquilizing effect on the body, unless too much is done too late in the day (later than 6 p.m.). When too much exercise is done too late in the evening, it temporarily increases the body's energy, which may make getting to sleep more difficult.

Spiritually speaking, any time we take care of ourselves, we are nurturing our inner Spirit. Regular exercise can provide kids with a sense of calm, joy, pride, motivation, accomplishment, and wellbeing. They will feel better about themselves as a person. As I wrote in the yoga section above, I believe that we cannot truly love and nurture others until we know how to love and nurture ourselves. Making time for regular exercise is a form of self-love and self-nurturing. We can teach and model this coping skill to our children, as a healthy way to take care of the self, so that the self can always be and do its best in the world.

Choosing The Right Exercise

Children do not have to go to a gym and "pump iron" for an hour, or "feel the burn" to get the health benefits of exercise. In fact, it is unhealthy for the body to overdo exercise. Too much exercise can actually weaken the body's immune functioning. Muscles can be pulled or sprained, or other parts of the body can be hurt from doing too much, too hard, too fast. Determining the intensity and amount of exercise that works best for you and your child is important. We are all unique. Experimenting with how long, how intense, how often, what time of day, and what types of activities your child enjoys will help you discover the combination that works best for you and your child.

Healthy exercise can be as simple as a bike ride; a walk, jog, or run around the neighborhood; rollerblading; jumping rope or jumping on a trampoline. For children, it could be playing a fun game of tag, chase or hide-n-seek outside with friends. If you enjoy the outdoors, taking a hike in a nearby park, going canoeing or kayaking, or riding in a paddleboat will do the trick. There are also many sports that can be done competitively or noncompetitively, such as baseball, basketball, football, volleyball, soccer, karate, cycling, swimming or bowling. Some people enjoy golf, tennis, table tennis ("ping-pong"), handball, or racquetball. It could be yoga, t'ai chi, aerobics, or "Sweating to the Oldies" with Richard Simmons.

The stores are filled with exercise books, videos and audio guides to select from. Any of these choices will get a person's blood circulating; bring in fresh, clean oxygen into the body and its organs; and give a gentle, stimulating massage to the internal organs so that they can do their job better. With regular exercise, you and your child can begin to feel less stressed, anxious, or depressed; more content, positive, and energetic; have more stamina; and experience an overall improvement in resiliency and physical health. Check out the list below for some easy exercise ideas.

30 Fun Ways To Get Exercise		
Ride a bike	Rollerblade or skate	Take martial arts
Take a walk	Jump rope	Walk the dog
Go for a jog	Go canoeing	Skip
Run	Go kayaking	Do cartwheels
Jump on a trampoline	Ice skate	Play table tennis
Play tag or chase	Ride a paddle boat	Shoot hoops
Play hide-n-seek	Take up a sport	Play catch
Take a hike at a park	Skateboard	Dance
Go bowling	Swim	Do Qigong
Take aerobics	Do yoga	Learn to rock climb
Join a gym class		

Breathing as a Form of Exercise

There is a breathing exercise with many health benefits that comes to us from Kundalini Yoga. It is called, the "Breath of Fire." Even though the air is pulled down deep into the body with this breath, it is considered short and shallow, rather than long and deep. Ravi Singh, whom I mentioned earlier in this chapter, teaches that "one minute of Breath of Fire in a pose or exercise, engenders internal effects that would have taken up to an hour with normal breathing." Note that Singh does not recommend the Breath of Fire for children younger than 16 years old because "it prematurely stimulates the sex and growth hormones in the pituitary gland." Instead, use long, deep breathing. The exercise below teaches how to do the Breath of Fire for older children.

> **Exercise:** To do the Breath of Fire, find a comfortable place to sit down with your spine straight. Close your eyes and your mouth, as this exercise is done through the nose. Begin by sniffing in once, as if you had a runny nose. There is very little force behind the sniff. Notice what your naval, abdomen, and diaphragm do when you sniff in. They should expand. Practice sniffing in until they expand when you sniff, even if you have to consciously make them expand at first. This means you are pulling the air down deep into your body. This is what you want. [If your abdomen contracts (or pulls in) when you sniff, you are pulling the air into your lungs.] When you have mastered the "inhale sniff", practice the "exhale sniff." This is the opposite action with the same amount of force. On the exhale sniff, your naval, abdomen, and diaphragm should contract (or pull in). If you concentrate on pulling your naval, abdomen, and diaphragm in on the exhale sniff, they will automatically expand on the inhale. So, to do the Breath of Fire, you sniff in and out in a rapid, shallow, gentle rhythm. The more you practice this breath, the easier and faster it will get for you. Remember, this is a shallow breath requiring very little force.

Singh says that practicing the Breath of Fire:

1. gives you the physical benefits of an aerobic workout without having to get your heart pumping rapidly;
2. helps keep fresh oxygen in the blood, which makes it easier for the body to detoxify itself;
3. puts the rhythms, systems, and organs of the body in sync;
4. gets the body's energy flowing;
5. warms you up when you are cold; and
6. when done on a regular basis, helps keep toxins out of the lungs.

All of these benefits help build the body's resilience and ability to regenerate itself. I have never felt anything uncomfortable when doing this breath, though Singh suggests that the first few times, your nose may sting or burn a bit. According to Singh, if you experience this, it "simply means that you are eliminating toxins via the nervous system." The breath is easy to learn, and you can get some benefit by practicing it as little as five minutes a day. Try it; you and your teen-ager may really like it.

Closing Thoughts on Exercise

No matter how you choose to get it, exercise is an important way to prevent health problems, reduce stress, increase vitality, and stay physically, mentally, emotionally and spiritually balanced. Most children enjoy exercise in the form of outdoor play, but some children will need support from their parents in making this a regular part of their life. Family activities can motivate children, and bring the family closer together. Many families enjoy walking or riding bicycles together. Some make regular trips to a roller or ice rink. Some go to a park for jungle gyms, hiking, and/or a picnic. A friendly game of softball, basketball, football, soccer, or catch will do. When playing for family fun and exercise, rules are unimportant (except for safety), and competition is generally not advised. The goal is simply to get everyone moving *and* having fun, so that you are all winners.

8

MODERN DAY HIGH-TECH LIVING

Digital technology's impact
on children's development

TODAY'S CHILDREN LIVE in a world that is full of high-tech gadgets that we have never had before as a society. For instance, they get a lot of entertainment from television, movies, computer and video games. Most have cell phones or pagers. Fax machines, personal computers (PCs), laptop computers and the World Wide Web ("www") are a fact of their lives, rather than a dream or a luxury. In managed doses, these forms of learning, fun and communication can be very useful and satisfying. They can help youngsters feel more connected to the society that they live in, and to their peer group. They can provide parents and children with a sense of safety and connection when they are away from each other. They can also connect youngsters to worlds that may be beyond their physical reach, but can be experienced in their imaginations or through the World Wide Web. They can even provide models of pro-social behavior, and support the development of certain skills, such as visual-spatial, critical thinking, and eye-hand coordination.

I have some concerns, however, about the effects of today's technology on certain aspects of children's development and behavior. This is especially true when access and use of these items is not well supervised. Although I recognize that this technology can be beneficial, I stand by the position that we need to move forward with caution in making these powerful "tools" available to our children.

Unlike mature adults, many children are not able to keep healthy limits on their use of these tools. Nor do they understand just how much of an influence the technology has on their lives.

This is a generation of "technological guinea pigs." As the first generation with access to all of this technology, we must learn what is healthy, and what is unhealthy; what is control, and what is responsibility; what is freedom, and what is abuse. We already know, however, positive from negative, compassionate from cold-hearted, tolerant from intolerant, responsible from irresponsible, and appropriate from inappropriate. As adults and parents, I believe that it is our duty to teach youngsters how to be positive, compassionate, tolerant, responsible and appropriate members of a society.

Although it is true that we are children's mentors, and that they learn from our behavior and our words, they also learn from what they experience in the environment. Do not be fooled into believing that our high-tech gadgets are safe for developing young psyches. That would be similar to allowing a preschooler to play with sharp scissors: there is plenty of room for danger if left unsupervised.

In this chapter, I address some of the ways that today's technology can negatively influence the psychological, emotional and behavioral functioning of our children. There is much more to this topic than I chose to discuss here, but to elaborate more is beyond the scope of this book. I did, however, want to raise your level of awareness about these issues, so that you can have an understanding of the impact they have on your child's behavior, and make educated decisions about what to allow into your child's world of experiences.

Virtual Reality, Virtual Life

Consider this reality: In the late 1990s, a group of junior high school students that I worked with thought that cable TV was one of their household "utility" bills. To them, this meant that it was as essential for their families as water or electricity. They did not know life without it, or a microwave, or a computer, or video games, or walkmans, or pocket-sized gadgets of all kinds, or cellular phones and pagers. This was *not* my experience growing up. I remember being outside visiting with friends and neighbors. I remember climbing into large trees and hanging out up there, watching. I watched the birds, people going by, bugs, leaves gently moving in the breeze, butterflies, and bees. I remember riding my bike, playing outdoor games, laughing, talking, reading or just sitting outside enjoying nature with friends, enjoying *life*. There were all kinds of entertaining things going on. In my youth, we entertained ourselves with *real* life, in *real* time, rather than with virtual life, in accelerated time.

Today, just about everything that many children spend their free time on is "virtual," meaning that it is modeled *after* real life, but it is *not* real life. They spend their recreational time absorbed in a virtual reality. In fact, many children (and adults, for that matter) are becoming more comfortable with "virtual life" than "real life." They experience it through TV, movies, computers, the Internet (the "net"), the World Wide Web (www.), and video and computer games of all types. They would rather "speak" to someone by typing on the computer (email) than calling him or her on the telephone. Chances are that even if they did call them on the telephone, they would be just as likely to get an answering machine or voicemail box as a real person.

There is more to this growing attraction to virtual life than meets the eye. Let us look at this issue more closely. Some of the most popular sites on the Internet are "chat rooms," singles sites, pornographic or sexual sites, and hate sites. Why is that? Although there is no scientific research that looks at this phenomenon, I can make some educated guesses based on common sense and psychology.

To understand this better, I turn to Humanistic Psychologist Abraham Maslow's Theory of Motivation. Maslow's Theory was proposed in the early 1940s and continues to be widely accepted as a basis for understanding much of human behavior. In this theory, Maslow suggested that the need for belonging, acceptance and love was second only to basic survival and safety needs, as a drive of human behavior. Next comes the need for esteem and respect; and lastly, what he called "self-actualization" or fulfilling what you believe to be your purpose in life.

When we look closely at virtual reality - whether it is through the net, computer and video games, TV or movies - we see that *anything* can be experienced there. Children can strive to fulfill their motivational drives through virtual reality. They can experience them actively, as a player in the game, or passively as an observer of a movie. Whether their participation is active or passive, however, they can identify with the characters enough to take on their traits, achievements and failures. They can be a hero or a villain. They can achieve dreams and goals. They can attain power and respect, or find love and acceptance. These are things that we strive for in real life, and either fear losing once we achieve them, or fear failing in our attempts. But in virtual reality, these things can be experienced without worrying about consequences, creating a safer arena to "live in." Let's look more deeply at this idea.

Safety through anonymity. In virtual reality, the fear factor does not exist. So, if a child fails at a computer or video game, they can simply hit a reset button and do it over again. If their beloved TV or movie character fails, it does not affect their real life in any lasting way. If they hurt someone's feelings, or someone hurts their feelings on the Internet, they never have to contact them again. They don't *really* know your child anyway. They only know who your child allowed them to know through their "chats." You see, these virtual realities create a sense of safety that does not exist in the real world – a psychological, emotional, and behavioral safety. Kids feel they can do what they want without lasting consequences. They can be anonymous. When anonymous, it's easier for them to falsely believe that they are not accountable or responsible in any real way for their thoughts, emotions, or behavior.

Separation from the self. On another level, what the virtual reality experience creates is separation from the self. Rather than focusing on their own thoughts, feelings, and behaviors in real life, children can focus on the experiences of others through virtual reality. This is an easy way for them to avoid, or dissociate from, their real life situations. Real life experiences are much more challenging than are virtual experiences, because they demand our attention and action. If youngsters focus on real life, they may need to find a solution to a conflict, or take a long, deep look at themselves as a person. They may need to admit to a fault or faulty behavior. They might have to take a personal risk. These can all be very scary things to do.

In contrast, escaping to virtual reality is easy. Most humans will choose the "path of least resistance" (i.e., the easiest way through) in life, especially youth. So, virtual reality becomes the likely escape for a troubled or frightened youngster. The problem is that this escape may keep them from seeking the help and support they truly need in life, aside from bombarding their bodies with stimulation that can be energetically dark and heavy. It appears that this dynamic played a role in at least one of the school shootings that took place in the past decade – the Columbine school shootings in Colorado in 1999. Two students created a real-life shooting rampage at their high school, modeled after a video game, and left 12 students and a teacher dead, plus 24 others wounded, before killing themselves.

Separation from others. To cope with real life, a child must be willing to deal with their own thoughts, feelings, and behaviors, and then, to look at how these affect the people around them. This means that first, they must be connected to themselves, and second, recognize their connection to others. Using virtual reality as an escape not only separates youngsters from themselves, but also has the potential to separate them from others.

Many children spend their time focused on virtual reality relationships, so that they can ignore or escape from real life relationships. This limits their real life experiences, which, in turn, can limit their ability to function in pro-social ways in the real world. This is not to say that children cannot learn from virtual reality experiences that provide a model of pro-social behavior. They certainly can. Eventually, however, they will have to apply the learned behavior to real life situations. The same is true for antisocial models of behavior. Children can learn aggression, violence, and cruelty from virtual reality experiences, and then, can apply them to real life situations (which is what happened in the Columbine shooting).

Most of the computer games on the market are about winning. They foster competition and an "every man for himself" attitude. This is a form of social modeling that kids will absorb into their psyches. How many times have you heard a child (if not your own) parrot a line of defiance from a movie or TV show they've seen? The characters in TV shows, movies and games can serve as cultural role models to kids, who copy their language, dress and behavior in their struggles to explore and establish identity. When they participate in too much virtual reality, the lines between life "out here" and life "in there" – in their virtual reality world – can begin to blur and overlap in unhealthy ways.

Speed, Over-Stimulation and AD/HD

There is no question that today's technology has created the fastest-paced and most over-stimulated society in history. Consider this quote from two licensed naturopathic physicians in Washington, Drs. Judyth Reichenberg-Ullman and Robert Ullman in their book, *Ritalin Free Kids*:

> "Children spend hours playing Nintendo rather than romping in the woods or playing outside. Many are glued to the television set. Movies are speedier, scarier, and more violent than ever before. There is a growing atmosphere of hurriedness, intensity, and urgency. We eat fast, play fast, and channel-surf...People look for caffeine and drugs of all kinds to make them go faster and stay up longer...Our society places little value on tranquility, quiet, solitude, and the simple joy of being in nature."[7]

Dr. Thomas Armstrong, author of *The Myth of the A.D.D. Child*, agrees, and believes that TV, movies, computer and video games contribute to the short attention spans of today's youth because of the "constant shifting of visual frames...so that the viewer's reference point shifts every few seconds." He writes that this type of rapid, intense stimuli sets children up to have symptoms that we associate with AD/HD:

> "By creating high-impact audio and visual information in short blasts, television (and video games) may be secretly undermining some natural attentional mechanisms in the human mind. Through the use of sudden close-ups, pans, zooms, bright colors, sudden noises, and other attention-

getting mechanisms, television programmers (and video game designers) may be reducing the child's natural vigilance, or ability to remain actively focused on events taking place in the real world. And since children who are having their "thrill and danger" centers constantly provoked by TV and video games are given no immediate context for responding,...this pent-up need for physical response can manifest as over-activity, frustration, or irritability."[8]

Games for youngsters on the market today are louder, smaller (mobile), faster, more realistic, more sexual, more violent, and more stimulating to the senses than ever before. We now have a generation with many youth who have spent much of their free time being "entertained" by these virtual realities. In doing so, they can experience any of the following:

1. cruelty, aggression, and violence for a reward;
2. separation of self from feelings, and from others and their feelings;
3. desensitization, or a loss of compassion;
4. disconnection or dissociation from reality;
5. a self-centered and egotistical world view; and
6. heightened feelings of aggression, fear and anxiety.

They may also be learning antisocial problem-solving skills - and enjoying it - through these virtual reality experiences. I believe we have a situation on our hands as a society that demands swift action for change. Many painful events have occurred recently among our youth that serve as a "wake up" call, including some of the school shootings across the nation that have been associated with video game and movie images. We can safely say that something is missing in the lives of our youth when they model the destructive and unhealthy images and ideas they see on a movie or video screen, instead of reaching out for help in the real world from the people who love them.

Dr. Richard DeGrandpre, a Psychology Professor and author of the book *Ritalin Nation*, suggests that children are experiencing sensory addictions based on our "rapid-fire" culture. He theorizes that children's brains adjust and adapt to the pace or speed of their surroundings. In today's world of fast-paced, instant everything, children's brains get addicted to the intensity of the stimulation they are exposed to from movies, TV, videos, games, and computer activities. Symptoms of anxiety and restlessness surface in situations where the same level of stimulation is not available. To counter the uneasy feeling that develops, children search for ways to recreate a similar level of stimulation in their surroundings. This addiction, paired with weaker family structures that no longer provide children with a strong external framework, have resulted in behavioral shifts that we label as AD/HD, for example. There is a lot of truth to this theory.

We wonder why so many children are hyperactive, impulsive and inattentive? Think about the emotional experiences, training, practice and learning that so many of them are exposed to every day through modern technology and virtual reality. Let me venture to review some of the lessons youngsters learn from the modern technology they are exposed to:

1.	Fast is best, and the faster the better.
2.	I want things *now*; I should not have to wait.
3.	My wishes are more important than anyone else's.
4.	Other people are not important, especially if they keep me from what I want.
5.	I must be the most powerful and the strongest to succeed.
6.	I do not care if I hurt others in working toward my goals.
7.	It's an "everyone for themselves" world.
8.	I can handle things on my own, without support from others.
9.	If it isn't fast, colorful, loud, and/or in constant motion, it is boring.
10.	If I don't "win", I'm a loser.

These subtle messages are forces that can create trauma, chaos, discomfort, and fear on a very deep, subconscious - or even unconscious - level of being that will not simply disappear once the screen is turned off. These are messages that can linger in your child's body, psyche and being forever. It is my belief that when a youngster absorbs these kinds of forces or energies, they contribute to the development of emotional responses like the ones seen with the symptoms of AD/HD and other mental or emotional "disorders." I believe that it is time for us to step out of our passive sense of security around today's technology, and make aware and thoughtful choices about what we allow our children to be exposed to.

Speed And Instant Gratification

Modern society does not want to wait for *anything* - not for a busy telephone line to clear or for a letter to make its way through the postal delivery system. In my view, the fact that the postal service system is now called "snail mail" is one sign of how far away we have gotten from a slower, more natural pace of things in the world. For many people, especially children, this speedy, artificial reality we have created through technology is what they know and desire. Faster is viewed as best, and the faster, the better.

This quick access to everything (speed) is inescapable in today's world. Microwave ovens, fax machines and computers have helped to shift "real" time to "instant" or "virtual" time - we want it right here, right now. We have our own VCRs to watch movies whenever we want. We have cellular phones to talk to people whenever we want. We have our own computers, portable computers, and the World Wide Web so that we can do what we want, when we want, where we want - all in record time. We don't have to wait for anyone or anything. We have everything we want right at our fingertips in our own home or wherever we happen to be. We have (and are learning to *expect*) instant communication and instant satisfaction. We get annoyed if we have to wait in line or on hold. We have come to believe that our desires take priority over most everything else. This situation has created a generation of youth that does not have to wait for *anything* in a typical day - except maybe until the end of a school day to get home to their gadgets. And we wonder why kids seem so impatient and bored these days? Just look around at the training that is a major part of their "virtual" lives every day. How can real life (or life based on the pace of nature) compare to that kind of extreme?

This virtual world of high energy and speed that technology has created (and successfully marketed) is, in my view, the downfall of many youngsters in this generation. Not only do these technologies have the potential to create impatience, intolerance and separation from self and others by way of producing separation from reality, but many of them have the potential to promote antisocial behaviors like violence, sexualizing, greed, and a completely self-centered world view. Let's take a closer look at how technology can negatively influence children's behavior.

Virtual Violence And Antisocial Behavior

Some people claim that playing computer and video games is no different from watching television and movies, but the truth is that they are very different. With TV and movies, people participate by watching and listening only. You do not actually do anything. This is considered a "passive learning experience." Yet, your mind is very active, taking in information, ideas, and values from what you see. Research shows that after watching violence on television, people's aggressive behavior grows by 3 to 15 percent. There is also evidence showing that homicides and aggression increase in areas where there are televisions in the homes. Keep in mind that we remember 20% of what we hear, 30% of what we see, and 50% of what we see and hear (such as with TV and movies).

With computer and video games, however, youngsters are watching, listening, *and* doing. This is considered an "active learning experience." Whereas we remember 50% of what we see and hear, we remember 70% of what we say and 90% of what we say and do. How many times have you witnessed a youngster playing a computer or video game, and they are yelling to their opponent in the game? Here are some examples of what I have heard: "I got you, sucker!" "Die!

Die! Die!" "You're going down!" "Loser!" "You want a piece of me?" "Come see what I've got!" In these situations, children are watching, listening, speaking, and doing violence.

Psychology tells us that every time our children play a game that involves cruelty or violence, they learn that this is good behavior through something known as "classic behavior modification" -- they get either a positive or negative response for their behavior in the game. For instance, players earn rewards for behavior that allows them to reach a goal (i.e., they win, which often means that their "opponent" loses or dies). Players are punished for behavior that fails to reach a goal (i.e., their virtual being fails, loses or dies). This is why virtual game experiences have a much deeper impact on people's psyches than TV or movies do. Not only do the players become a part of the experience, they *learn* from their behavior through a series of rewards and punishments.

In games that have cruel or violent themes, the more violent the player is, the more successful they are at the game. And since most of the games require more severe kinds of violence to move up through the game levels, youngsters learn to see violence as a positive problem-solving tool. Lieutenant Colonel Grossman, a military expert on the psychology of killing, once said that "every time a child plays a point-and-shoot video game, he (or she) is learning the exact same conditioned reflex skills as a soldier or police officer in training." He also stressed that in playing games with cruel or violent themes, youngsters are learning to kill, and are learning to like it. Is this a lesson we want our children and youth to learn and carry with them into adulthood?

Besides becoming more likely to be aggressive and harmful to others from playing virtual games with cruel, violent or aggressive themes, youngsters are also learning other antisocial behaviors. For example, they may become less sensitive to the pain and suffering of others. They may be more anxious and fearful of the world around them, and develop mistrust of others. They may have poor self-confidence about their academic abilities and acceptance by peers. They may show more anger and hostility toward others. In fact, certain movies and video games are now seen as having played a part in at least some of the school shootings that have taken place in the last three years. For these reasons, it is so very important for caregivers (parents, grandparents, relatives, babysitters, etc.) to monitor and supervise youngster's TV viewing, and computer and video game playing, as much as possible. As Lt. Col. Grossman said: "If we had a clear-cut objective of raising a generation of assassins and killers who are unrestrained by either authority or the nature of the victim, it is difficult to imagine how we could do a better job."

Closing Thoughts on Technology

I recognize that today's technology has a positive place in our world. It is not necessarily the technology that is harmful, but the way we use it, or allow it to be used. Children's psyches are vulnerable. Premature exposure to the negative messages and energies that are a part of the technology world can affect them on a deep level. We cannot always see the effects outwardly, but we can be certain that they are impacting them inwardly.

Remember the standard parental saying, "As long as you are living under my roof...?" As a parent, it is your right *and* your obligation to check everything your child exposes their psyche to. When allowed in small, *positive-energy* doses, high-tech entertainment can have a beneficial influence on your child's development. Consider limiting and monitoring their use of this type of fun, rather than eliminating it. Find movies, games, videos, etc., that teach something of value to your child, and provide "clean," fun entertainment.

9

BALANCING THE BODY AND THE BRAIN

Ways to align them without drugs

BEFORE THE EXISTENCE of hospitals and pharmacies, there were healers who used the natural medicines of the Earth, along with the energies of the physical, mental, emotional and spiritual/energetic bodies, to treat symptoms. They worked with the rhythms of nature, under-standing how much power is found within the natural flow of life—the loving and creative energy that flows through us, surrounds us and binds us all together. They recognized that to try to move against the natural flow meant certain resistance and likely failure.

This is no longer theory. Science has proven that there is a dynamic energy field in and around all things, including objects we perceive to be solid or non-living, like tables and rocks. It is called "life force" or "aura" by some. This is what the field of quantum physics stud-ies – the energy of life that can't be seen with our eyes, but that can be identified, felt and measured with special tools. And *every thing* has an energy field, because every thing is made up of nothing more than energy and space at its core. If we were to microscopically view the world, all we would see is one, dynamic, fluid field of energy – like an energy ocean – with billions of different "energy dances" going on between particles within the ocean…each particle separate, but part of the whole ocean of energy and space.

Those of us who have been born and raised in the Western world have not been educated about the energy that is life, or about the energy systems of the body, and so may feel less comfortable with these healing approaches than folks raised in or educated about Eastern healing methods. Yet, Eastern cultures have studied and used the energetic systems of the body successfully for health and healing for centuries. That is why Western doctors and scientists have begun to take notice in recent decades, and to learn more about these methods.

One system that has become more popular in the U.S. is the system of "chakras" or energy centers within the body that contribute to our life force, vitality and health. There are seven of them in the ancient system that originated in India, running from the base of the spine at the tailbone up to the top of the head, or crown. Each chakra center aligns with a different aspect of our energetic Being: from our Root – which is our sense stability and safety, to our Sacral area – which is our creativity, passion, sexuality, and life force, to our Solar Plexus – which is our will and sense of personal power, to our Heart – which is our openness and love, to our Throat – which is our truth, to our Third Eye – which is our intuition, to our Crown, which is our wisdom and sense of Oneness. When there is a block in one or more of these chakra centers, it affects the others, which affects the functioning of the body and Being in general. Working with the chakras is one way to bring the energetic aspect of our Being into alignment, as part of a holistic model of health.

In Eastern parts of the world, where holistic health has been a way of life for centuries, the energetic body is considered just as important to wellbeing and functioning as the mental, physical, emotional and spiritual bodies are. Working with the chakras is one way to clear the flow of energy within the body to raise vitality and wellbeing. Today, many Western doctors and healers believe that physical symptoms are a sign of a blockage in the energy systems of the body. Biophysical methods of healing can open the blocked areas, balance the body's energy fields, bring back the natural flow of the systems, and help the body work as harmoniously as it is created to. Oftentimes, this simple solution of opening up and harmonizing energetic flow within the main systems and organs of the body – the brain, heart, circulatory system, nervous system and structural system, which then communicate with every muscle, organ and cell – can support it in healing and balancing itself.

Biophysics is the science of applying physical methods to biological issues. It works by opening flow between the physical and energetic systems of the body. In the case of children's health, there are many ways to use biophysical healing methods to calm behavioral symptoms. Of the many biophysical healing methods that are available, I will discuss five in this section: Biofeedback (or "neurofeedback"), Chiropractic Care, CranioSacral therapies, Acupuncture and Pediatric Tuí na, and links between Sensory Input (Vision Therapy, Sensory Scrambling, and Sensory Integration) and symptoms of AD/HD. I selected these five areas because they have been scientifically and/or clinically researched and noted to reduce the symptoms we call AD/HD for many people. Let's start with biofeedback.

Biofeedback

What is Biofeedback?

Biofeedback therapies were created in the 1970s as a way to work with the body's natural signals. The process of biofeedback involves having sensors attached to the skin with conductive paste, usually on a finger, on the chest, scalp, abdomen or ear, around the nose or mouth, or on a certain area of muscle. When the body responds physically to a certain signal or brain wave, the audio and visual information you get from the biofeedback machine lets you voluntarily change your brain waves and/or control the response of your body. Basically, you learn how to control the kind of brain waves that your body produces or the physiological response that your body has, to a pattern that will help you the most in a given situation. Any change in your body that can be measured can be used for biofeedback.

There are six common types of measurements used in biofeedback. They are:

1. Electroencephalographic (EEG) Neurofeedback, which records brain waves (or brain electricity) so that you can see them, know them, and control them better;

2. Electromyographic (EMG) feedback, which measures muscle tension so you can learn to relax or tense certain muscles as needed;

3. Thermal feedback, which measures skin temperature as a gauge of constricted blood flow so you can learn to reduce this in the hands and feet. Restricted blood flow could signal changes in the reflexes of the nervous system;

4. Electroderman Activity (EDA), which measures changes in sweat activity as an index of changes in the reflexes of the nervous system so that you can practice relaxation;

5. Finger Pulse, which measures pulse rate and force (the amount of blood in each pulse) to check for heart activity that may mean arousal of part of the nervous system; and

6. Breathing, in which breath rate, volume, rhythm, and location (chest or abdomen) are measured and recorded so you can learn to pull more air down deeper, slower, and more rhythmically.

Some biofeedback therapists may use what is called a "skull cap." This involves putting a swimming-type cap on the head that has 19 electrodes in it to measure the responses of certain parts of the brain. These sensors measure brain wave frequencies and amplitudes that are then given to the person through audio and visual feedback. There are five kinds of brain waves that are produced with different activities:

1. Delta waves when sleeping deeply;

2. Theta waves when deeply relaxing or meditating;

3. Alpha waves when day dreaming, calm, unfocused, and relaxed;

4. Sensorimotor rhythm waves when calm, still, quiet, and alert;

5. And Beta waves when thinking and concentrating.

Is Biofeedback Safe?

The instruments used for biofeedback are safe and cannot shock you. The treatment is painless, gentle, and there are no side effects. It seems to produce lifelong results. The Association for Applied Psychophysiology and Biofeedback recommends that anyone with a severe heart disorder or with an implanted electrical device (such as a pacemaker) ask their doctor before trying biofeedback. Also, talk to your doctor about wanting to try biofeedback, and if your child is taking medications, be sure and report them to the biofeedback therapist, since drugs prescribed for the AD/HD diagnosis alter brain activity.

Is Biofeedback Effective?

Biofeedback therapy is used with both children and adults. It can work well with other therapies (such as relaxation training) for dealing with headaches, stress, anxiety, and muscle tension. Biofeedback has been used in the treatment of the AD/HD diagnosis since irregular brain wave patterns have been found in those with the symptoms. Here, one theory is that the brain produces too few beta-waves (used for concentration, focusing, paying attention, staying on task, thinking sequentially, comprehension, and understanding cause and effect) and too many alpha-waves (linked to inattention, distractibility, "spaciness," poor memory, disorganization, poor task sequencing, and daydreaming). Biofeedback can be used to bring brainwave functioning back into balance.

Research using topographic (EEG) brain-mapping shows this difference does exist in individuals diagnosed with AD/HD. We just do not know what causes the difference. A research review of studies that evaluated the usefulness of biofeedback as a component of treating AD/HD-like symptoms concluded that it does have a positive effect. Biofeedback may result in higher intelligence scores, academic gains, positive social behaviors, and fewer behavioral and cognitive difficulties. The review also showed that biofeedback, in combination with a new technique known as Instantaneous Neuronal Activation Procedure (INAP), resulted in quicker results.

Other research shows that glucose metabolism in the brains of adults who were diagnosed with AD/HD as children was abnormally low, especially in the areas that control attention and motor activity. This goes back to the idea that the symptoms might be related to a neuro-metabolic problem, which involves nutrition and the metabolism as described in Chapter 6. With biofeedback, patients learn how to reverse these patterns using the machine, and then to eventually create the same effect without the machine. Of course, we do not know the role that medication played in these findings (since subjects had used the drugs). There is research showing that many people have had success with biofeedback, and have been able to stop using other treatments like drugs. Research also shows that the effects of this technique lasts for many, many years after the therapy ends. There is no way to say the change is "permanent," because research subjects are not typically followed until death.

One study done by Dr. Thomas Rossiter and Dr. Theodore LaVaque compared the effects of stimulant drugs to biofeedback, along with other treatments. The results showed that biofeedback training led to major drops in the mental and behavioral symptoms of children diagnosed with AD/HD after 20 treatments over just 4 to 7 weeks. Reports from mothers and from tests done to measure certain behaviors showed that there were great improvements in attention, impulse control, speed of information processing, and consistency of attention. The results also showed that symptoms of psychopathology lessened. These changes were noticeable outside of the testing setting and in the children's daily lives. Rossiter and LaVaque claim that their results are equal to those achieved with drugs, and are the same as results reported from other research in this field.

Dr. Siegfried Othmer and Susan Othmer are researchers and certified neurofeedback practitioners who have done extensive work with people diagnosed with AD/HD. Their research suggests that biofeedback works by strengthening the brain's natural ability to regulate itself. Essentially, the brain is given time to practice and strengthen a skill that other children's brains naturally do well. Once the mastery has taken place, the brain will keep using the skill, and it will continue to improve. The Othmers reported several positive outcomes from their work using biofeedback training for the symptoms of AD/HD. These include:

1.   children could more easily access and use their natural mental capabilities;

2.   visual and auditory retention skills improved (children were better able to remember what they saw and heard);

3.   children could concentrate better;

4.   reading, math, enunciation, and verbal expression skills improved;

5.   handwriting, motor skills, and coordination improved;

6.   handedness regulated (children began to use one or the other);

7.   grades improved;

8.   self-esteem increased;

9.   hyperactivity decreased;

10. organization improved;

11. children slept better, were less irritable, had fewer headaches, and fewer food sensitivities; and

12. results lasted between 6 and 9 months after the training.

These are significant findings because they suggest that biofeedback training can benefit the physical, mental, *and* emotional aspects of a child's functioning. Rather than masking symptoms the way drugs do, biofeedback appears to *teach* a life-changing skill to children.

Dr. Thomas Armstrong reported on findings from a research review of biofeedback completed by Steven Lee of the University of Kansas. This review shows that when used with other therapies, biofeedback does seem to reduce some of the symptoms of hyperactivity. Dr. Joel Lubar, a psychologist at the University of Tennessee who first developed this treatment, claims that the use of biofeedback training has allowed many children to decrease or stop using their medication for hyperactivity. Laura Stevens, a researcher in the field of nutrition and AD/HD, reports in her book, *12 Effective Ways to Help Your ADD/*

ADHD Child that "on the average, attention and concentration improve, organizational skills develop, and the child is less impulsive and hyperactive." Research shows that other improvements may be seen in ability to focus, school grades, task completion, behavior and learning skills, social skills, intelligence test scores, handwriting, eye-hand coordination, math skills, problem solving, bed-wetting, speech difficulties, self-esteem, and job performance. These are pretty impressive results to think about.

What to Consider With Biofeedback

Dr. Thomas Armstrong listed guidelines for parents who are considering biofeedback for their child. These include:

1. It is best viewed as an addition to other treatments instead of thinking that it will solve all the problems on its own;

2. Do not trust claims of "100% cures" or miraculous changes from biofeedback; it is a very individual process;

3. It may not be OK for children who are dealing with depression, seizures, psychotic episodes or who are younger than 7 years;

4. Choose an experienced, clinically certified biofeedback practitioner who has lots of experience working with attention problems;

5. Remember that the child makes the changes, not the machine; the machine is just a way to get the changes started.

One drawback to biofeedback is that it is generally expensive and time-consuming. Initial screenings can cost more than one hundred dollars, with anywhere from 6 to 50 follow-up sessions that last from 40 to 50 minutes each at a cost of between $60 and $150 per session. This may put it out of reach for some people, although there are some insurance companies that reimburse for biofeedback. Check with yours to see what they might cover. Success is reported for 80% of the patients when they are properly screened, but there are no guarantees. Still, if you can afford the time and money needed for this treatment, you may find that any lasting and far-reaching benefits are well worth it.

If you decide to try bio- (or neuro) feedback, there are some organizations that you can contact for more information. Susan Othmer is the Executive Director of the E.E.G. Spectrum Institute in Los Angeles, California. Currently, they have over 200 affiliated offices in 43 states in the U.S. Visit their website to find a clinic in your area. For example, there are several clinics in Texas, including four in Austin; two in Corpus Christi, Houston, and San Antonio; and one in Plano and Round Rock. The E.E.G. Spectrum Institute can be contacted by phone at 1-800-789-3456, or by writing or calling:

E.E.G. Spectrum Institute
16500 Ventura Boulevard, Suite 418
Encina, California 91436-2505
PHONE: 1-818-788-2083
FAX: 1-818-728-0933
www.eegspectrum.com

Choosing a Biofeedback Specialist

Finding the best biofeedback therapist for your child may take a bit of research. Here are some guidelines to help you with your search:

1. Get referrals (names of biofeedback therapists) from people you know and trust if possible. In Texas, you can contact the Biofeedback Society of Texas at (512)328-9639 for information.

2. Contact the therapist and ask as many questions as you need to for your comfort; a good therapist will happily answer all of them to your satisfaction (as long as they have the time).

3. Check their licensure and training:
   - Find out what academic degrees they have.
   - Find out what licensure they have. Ideally, they will have a license from the Biofeedback Certification Institute of America (BCIA), but this is not necessary for them to be an able practitioner.

4. Look for a therapist who:
   - is an independent practitioner (they can practice without supervision) or is supervised by a licensed practitioner;
   - has been practicing for at least 2 years;
   - has experience working with children.

5. Be sure you feel safe and comfortable with the therapist. You want to trust what they do with your child. If you do not feel comfortable with something the therapist says or does, talk to them about it. Be willing to try another therapist if one does not work out for you.

Chiropractic Therapy

What Is It?

Chiropractic therapy is a method of healing that focuses on the functioning of the central nervous system. The central nervous system runs from your head down to your toes. Every action that your body performs is in some way related to the signals of the central nervous system. The theory behind chiropractic therapy is that disease results from abnormal functioning of the nerves in some area of the body. Blockages to the signals of the central nervous system generally result from misalignments of the body's bone structure. These misalignments cause "kinks" in the surrounding soft tissues that connect and bind the body's structure together, such as the muscles, tendons, fascia, and nerves. When the body's bone structure is realigned, nerve functioning is restored and the symptoms improve and may disappear altogether.

Chiropractic treatment focuses on making adjustments to the soft tissue and/or skeletal structure of the body in a specific area thought to be out of alignment and obstructing nerve functioning. This is achieved through either manual manipulations or the use of machines. Manual manipulations are the adjustments that chiropractors do to the neck, spine, or any other area of the body where bones are found to be out of alignment. Many chiropractors also use electrical or other devices to stimulate the muscles or stretch out the spinal column. The goal is to keep the body in perfect alignment so that the nervous system can function properly.

Chiropractic therapy has long been practiced as an "alternative" health care approach for its benefits to the spinal column and central nervous system. As a healing art, it has only recently begun to make its way into mainstream modern medicine (and be covered by some insurance policies). Chiropractors became "famous" for treating whiplash victims. Most of us know that if we are involved in even a mild car accident, we may need to see a chiropractor to address neck or back pain afterwards. Time has shown, however, that the art of chiropractic care has many other benefits. Treating the symptoms linked to AD/HD is one area that is coming to the forefront in this field.

Is It Safe?

From the information that I reviewed about chiropractic therapy, and from my personal experiences with it, I can say that it is generally safe. It is important to choose a therapist who is properly licensed to practice this method. You will find suggestions for choosing a chiropractor at the end of this chapter.

Although I did not find research about the safety of chiropractic methods, I also did not find any articles that discussed problems from the therapy. Personally, I chose to change chiropractors once, following a standard adjustment to my neck that left me with a pulled muscle down my back. I had been working with this particular chiropractor for years without any problems. I'm not certain what happened on that day, but I took it as a sign that my body no longer wanted that type of adjusting. I still work with a chiropractor, specifically, an upper cervical chiropractor, and have not had any problems. The adjustments done by upper cervical chiropractors involve an extremely mild (in fact, I barely feel anything) manipulation of the Atlas Plate, rather than the typical "cracking" of the spinal bones that traditional chiropractors use. Keep in mind that children's bodies are much more flexible than adults', so they will adjust more readily. Chiropractors who work with children are generally sensitive to their special needs.

Is It Effective?

As with other healing methods, chiropractic treatment and treatment outcomes are very individual. The type of chiropractic care that will work best for someone depends on their personal history and profile. According to the research, it appears that chiropractic methods focusing on the upper cervical area, as well as specific sites on the spinal column, can both be effective for reducing symptoms of AD/HD in children. I review some of this research below.

Chiropractic Therapy as Treatment for Symptoms of AD/HD

Chiropractic care has shown up strongly in recent times for the treatment of symptoms related to AD/HD. There is research suggesting that better results can be achieved with chiropractic care than with medication. For example, Garber and his colleagues reported in their book, *Beyond Ritalin,* success with an approach called, "neural organization technique," which is based on the idea that the symptoms of AD/HD are due to a misalignment of certain parts of the skull and spine. Supporters of this procedure claim that spinal adjustments can correct the misalignment and resolve the symptoms.

Consider also the work of Robert Goodman, Doctor of Chiropractic and member of the National Upper Cervical Chiropractic Association (NUCCA). Dr. Goodman wrote an article sharing his experiences with treating AD/HD patients at his office in Boulder City, Nevada. He explained that the Atlas Plate is the part of the neck located at the base of the skull where the head and neck meet. When the Atlas Plate is "knocked out" of its proper placement in the neck, it causes the alignment between the head and the neck to be lost. The result is contracted muscles in the spine, and restriction of the nerves at the brain stem level, which keeps the muscles and nerves of the central nervous system from working correctly. This is referred to as "Atlas Subluxation Complex." In time, as the body tries to compensate for the misalignment, the problems can actually get worse. In Dr. Goodman's practice, patients with an Atlas Subluxation Complex, who also have a diagnosis of AD/HD, experience fewer symptoms of AD/HD after treatment for the Atlas Subluxation Complex.

Dr. Patricia Gregg, a Doctor of Chiropractic and member of NUCCA with a clinical practice in Austin, Texas, explained to me that upper cervical spinal correction is "designed to restore body balance and reactivate the body's self-healing process." This is the case because *every* nerve in the body either starts, ends, or passes through the neck-spine junction of our bodies. The idea (very simply put) is that if something happens to move the Atlas Plate even slightly off center, the spine below the head will try to deal with the "tilt" by shifting into abnormal positions. This leads to pressure at the brainstem level, which the atlas surrounds, disrupting the messages that come and go from the brain to control the rest of the body. Although these changes may not be visible to the untrained eye, many different symptoms can follow, including nervous tension, loss of sleep, fatigue, headaches, light-headedness or dizzy spells, depression, child development problems, hypertension, muscle spasms, nervousness, and aches and pains of different body parts, to name a few. When the tilt is gently corrected and the body is given time to readjust itself to a normal (or balanced) position, the symptoms begin to go away, and usually stay away.

To further complicate this issue, consider that there is research showing that the birth process itself can result in subluxations. More than 80 pounds of pressure is typically applied by doctors to an infant's head and neck during the birth process. This is enough to cause subluxations in the necks of infants at birth. In a seminar entitled, "Complimentary Drug-Free Treatments for Symptoms of ADD/ ADHD," Dr. Dan Powers explained that "the pushing, pulling, and twisting on the newborn's neck and spine during birth commonly causes the small vertebrae to be pushed out of place...Throughout life, falls, injuries, and stress commonly cause subluxations. Young children may fall down several times a day, a common occurrence that, along with contact sustained in sports activities, may cause vertebrae to move out of their natural alignment." He has been a chiropractor for about 20 years and owns "Powers Family Chiropractic" in Austin, Texas. This view is supported by the fact that more boys than girls are diagnosed with AD/HD, knowing that in general, boys tend to play harder than girls, and therefore, are more likely to have subluxations.

Dr. Powers said that in his practice, more and more children are turning up who have no curve in their neck, or a reversed curve. These situations begin with subluxations to the neck and spine which, when untreated, evolve into serious misalignments. When there is subluxation in the bones of the back, the nerves become twisted or stretched, and communication between the brain and the nerves is disrupted. Subluxation disrupts this flow because proper alignment of the vertebrae is what allows the brain signals to filter down the spinal cord to the nerves. Since the entire body is run by the brain in communication with the nerves, neurological, emotional, and physical symptoms or disorders result. Some of the symptoms that Dr. Powers noted are perceptual problems, poor posture, poor flexibility in the neck, and many symptoms related to AD/HD (such as distractibility and over-activity).

Keep in mind that only 10% of the central nervous system is considered "pain sensitive." This means that there can be a problem in some part of the system that shows up in "soft signs" (such as confusion, distractibility, over excitability, poor memory, etc.) rather than "hard signs" (such as pain in some part of the body). This makes it difficult to identify when something may be wrong in the body's alignment. A standard chiropractic exam can rule out the possibility that your child is dealing with a subluxation.

It is interesting to note that some chiropractors believe that the spine is a "shock organ," meaning that the bones in the spine move slightly out of their normal place when exposed to pollutants such as chemicals, food additives and preservatives, or dyes. Studies about this idea began in the 1950s, and are getting some support from more recent research.

For example, in an article printed in *Today's Chiropractic*, a professional journal for chiropractors, Dr. Webster reported his research findings on children diagnosed with AD/HD. He believes that the spine is indeed a shock organ, and that certain preservatives, dyes, and sugars caused abnormal readings of the spine as measured by nerve and thermal instruments, and palpation (examination by touch). Some changes could be found immediately after a child ate the suspected food.

Additionally, Dr. Powers explained that many food additives and artificial flavorings, for example, are considered neurotoxins because they wear off the protective sheath around the nerve strands, which impairs their ability to function. In my view, these are significant findings that could provide an important link between the symptoms seen in AD/HD and diet as it affects the body.

My personal experience with chiropractic care has involved both general chiropractic adjustments and treatment by a member of the National Upper Cervical Chiropractic Association (NUCCA). I worked with a general Doctor of Chiropractic off-and-on during my very early 30s for neck problems related to minor accidents and stress. This therapy provided some relief for my symptoms. Then, at age 34, I was involved in a high-impact, head-on car collision that resulted in various injuries, and problems with my neck, spine, and shoulders. After two years of chronic neck and back pain following the accident, a friend suggested that I switch to an NUCCA chiropractor.

My subsequent recovery was amazing to me. After only one "adjustment" in one year (with regular check-ups), I became virtually symptom-free. For example, I no longer had migraine headaches, light-headedness, dizzy spells, or chronic pain and fatigue. My ability to concentrate and focus for long periods of time returned. I could think more clearly and make decisions with less difficulty. My mood, attitude, and general outlook on life improved. I felt less tense and more relaxed. The treatment was so gentle that it is a wonder to me that anything at all shifted. It has been several years and my positive recovery has continued. I cannot guarantee that the results will be the same for everyone; I can only share that for me, they have been very positive.

What to Consider With Chiropractic Care

The cost of chiropractic care can vary dramatically from one practitioner to another. However, the cost of the initial evaluation can range from $150 to $400, and follow-up care is typically between $40 and

$100 per session. This may or may not include the cost of X-rays, or the use of special treatment machines, such as muscle stimulators (which activate and relax specific muscles) or Spinalators (a type of rolling bed that stretches out the spinal column). How long each treatment session lasts, and how many are needed, can only be determined on an individual basis. It will depend on the severity of the problem and the intensity of the treatment program. Generally, it may take 1 to 6 months to see lasting results. Many insurance companies are now paying for a limited number of chiropractic visits when prescribed by a doctor. Check with your insurance company for their criteria and coverage.

As with other therapies, there are no guarantees that all of your child's symptoms will improve with general or upper cervical chiropractic treatment. It is a very individual experience. Chiropractic care can, however, be a good compliment to other strategies or therapies you may employ. In my opinion, the research and testimonial data in support of this treatment suggests that it holds promise for at least some children with symptoms of AD/HD.

Choosing a Chiropractor

When searching for a chiropractor to treat your child, use the same general guidelines listed above for finding a biofeedback therapist:

1. Get referrals (names of chiropractors) from people you know and trust.

2. Contact the therapist and ask as many questions as you need to for your comfort; a good therapist will happily answer all of them to your satisfaction (as long as they have the time).

3. Check their licensure and training:
   - Find out what academic degrees they have;
   - Look for a Doctor of Chiropractic (DC), state and/or national licensure, and/or specialized training or membership (e.g., National Upper Cervical Chiropractic Association, Texas Chiropractic Association, American Chiropractic Association).

4. Look for a doctor who:
   - can practice independently (without supervision);
   - has been practicing for more than 3 years; and
   - has experience working with children.

5. Be sure you feel safe and comfortable with what the doctor is doing for your child. If you do not feel comfortable with something they say or do, talk to them about it. Be willing to make a change if it does not work for you.

CranioSacral Therapy

What Is It?

CranioSacral Therapy (CST) is considered an "off-shoot" of chiropractic therapy. Like chiropractic therapy, it involves gentle adjustments that are made with the hands of a trained therapist. The difference is that CranioSacral therapy focuses on adjusting the CranioSacral system of the body, specifically. The CranioSacral system includes the brain and spinal cord; the cerebrospinal fluid that surrounds the brain and spinal cord; the membranes that enclose the brain, spinal cord, and cerebrospinal fluid; and the bones of the spine and skull that hold the membranes. The pressure used is hardly noticeable, yet it directly affects the central nervous system.

Dr. Arturo Volpe, who is not only a Certified Nutritionist and Fellow with the International Academy of Medical Acupuncture, but also a Doctor of Chiropractic, uses CST at his health clinic in Houston, Texas. He explained that the skull is not one solid bone, but rather, is made up of several sections of bone that can shift slightly out of place after a blow to the head or other situations. The job of the therapist is to find where the shifts have occurred within the CranioSacral system and gently "manipulate" the bones back into their proper positions. This allows the brain and body to function normally again. In other words, balance will be restored to the body's energy systems (physical, mental, emotional, and spiritual/energetic), enabling them to align and flow in a more centralized manner. Symptoms that resulted from any misalignment should improve.

A CranioSacral therapist can tell when the flow of energy patterns in the body is out of balance, and which parts of the body are reacting to the imbalance. They will typically hold their hands up to the bottoms of your feet, and then up to your shoulders, to "read" the flow of energy from your body. Then, they will gently place their fingers to some part of the CranioSacral system with extremely minimal pressure, and hold the position for as little as 5, or as long as 30, minutes, before moving to a different location. In my personal experience, CST created harmony among the energy systems of my body so that my physical healing happened faster and easier, and the gains lasted longer.

Is It Safe?

It is important to work with a trained professional who is licensed to do CranioSacral therapy. In general, though, the treatments used in CST are safe, have no unwanted side effects, are pain-free, and are very gentle. I am not aware of any reports of problems from this therapy. I encourage you to plan the session for the end of the day, since it is so relaxing and can leave your child feeling "giddy" or "spacey."

Is It Effective?

Research and reports from the doctors who use CST support it as a very promising treatment choice for the symptoms of AD/HD in certain people. There can be dramatic changes for children and adults that are long lasting and make a positive difference in their overall functioning.

For example, Dr. John Upledger, who is considered an expert in CST, believes that certain cases of AD/HD symptoms are caused by a "jamming of the skull forward on the neck" that is not noticeable to the untrained. When this problem is corrected, the children begin to behave more normally. His clinic has had tremendous success with treating hyperactive, autistic, and learning disabled children with CST. Dr. Arturo Volpe also reports success with CST for certain patients who suffer from the symptoms of AD/HD at his clinic.

What to Consider With CranioSacral Therapy

In my view, CranioSacral Therapy is worth checking into either on its own or as a compliment to other strategies you may be using with your child, such as behavioral management, nutritional changes, therapy, etc. It will not interfere with other therapies or treatments. Although simpler and less expensive than some of the other choices, it is not inexpensive, and most insurance companies will not cover it. I estimate that therapists generally charge between $50 and $100 per session. The number, length, and frequency of sessions a person will benefit from are determined by their individual needs and the professional opinion of the therapist.

Choosing a CranioSacral Practitioner

Just as with choosing other health care providers, you will want a CST that is properly licensed, has a few years of experience, and is well trained in the arts of this type of therapy. I prefer to get verbal referrals from friends or health care providers that I trust. You may find it helpful to contact the Upledger Institute Healthplex, at (561)622-4706, or the American Chiropractic Association for information and referrals to therapists or clinics in your area. The Internet has sites that can be useful in gathering this type of information as well. I have also included a few organizations in the resource guide at the back of this book.

Chinese Acupuncture And Tuí Na

Although methods of Chinese Medicine may seem crude or strange to many Americans, this is because we do not understand them, and they are not a normal part of our lives, as they are in China. In the past, these ancient healing therapies have not been supported by the allopathic medical community in this country or by the insurance companies. Now that more attention is being given to natural healing in general, these time-tested Chinese Medicine methods are gaining more respect in the US.

Dr. Tom Williams explains in his book, *The Complete Illustrated Guide to Chinese Medicine,* acupuncture and tuí na are based on a large "body of knowledge" established through observing and recording "the effect of needling specific points and areas of the body." Over a period of thousands of years, the Chinese developed an energetic model of the body, including maps of the strong energy flow systems, or meridians, in the body. Along these meridians are certain points of high access to the heart of the energy flow. Acupuncture and tuí na use these access points to create changes in the flow of the energy systems of the body.

Chinese Medicine and their model of our energetic body is based on five "substances:"

1. **Qi** (pronounced, "Chee"), which refers to the body's life force energy. This governs the day-to-day movement and activity of the body;

2. **Jing,** which is the body's essence. This governs the long-term development and growth of the body from prebirth to death;

3. **Blood,** which nourishes and moistens the body and mind, supporting Shen;

4. **Body Fluids,** which moisten and lubricate the body and its organs;

5. **Shen,** which is our consciousness. This keeps the mind sharp and alert.

These substances are not viewed as "things," but instead, are used to describe a process in which they work as a balanced and dynamic system. The Chinese call it the "dance of life." They are the flowing energies of life through the body.

The focus of Chinese acupuncture and tuí na is on:

- removing energy blocks that may exist along the pathways of natural energy flow (meridians); this is generally evident by external pain;
- restoring internal harmony to the energy systems; or
- a combination of both.

The result is even-flowing energy with a relaxed sense of aliveness, connection or even exhilaration, plus a stronger ability to cope with stress or distraction. This is the opposite of hyperactivity, which can be described as a lot of energy that has no place to go due to blocks in certain meridians in the body. The difference between these two states is seen as balanced (even-flowing) energy versus imbalanced (either blocked or overflowing) energy – "energy in focus" versus "energy out of focus." The key is to bring the body's energy systems into balance so that there is neither too much nor too little in any area. This process is said to affect, for example, the central nervous system, the immune system, the mental and emotional bodies, and the health of the organs.

Treating Symptoms With Acupuncture

An acupuncturist will begin by completing an interview with your child (and you) about how they are doing and feeling, including any symptoms they are having. They may observe their appearance closely, check their tongue, smell them, listen to them, or touch them to identify any tender areas on the body, sense temperature and skin condition, and check their pulses. After assessing the situation, they will discuss their approach with you and your child. Then, your child will be asked to lie down on a "bed" like the ones in doctor's offices, either fully clothed, unclothed, or in a special gown. For certain purposes, patients may be asked to sit up on the bed for the treatment. Finally, the acupuncturist will place the needles on specific and purposeful meridians (energy channels) along your child's body.

The number of needles used each time will depend on your child's needs. Once the needles are set, your child will be allowed to rest undisturbed. Some acupuncturists will periodically "tweek" the needles by gently moving them while the patient is resting. This may create a tingly sensation. How long your child is allowed to rest, and whether their front, back, or both are treated, depends on the situation. Many people I know (including myself) who have used acupuncture tell me that they fall into a deep, relaxing sleep during the treatment. I have even had a dream or two.

Acupuncture needles are thinner than a piece of hair, so the treatments are generally pain-free. Sometimes, there may be a quick "sting" when a needle is set that may be due to a severe energy block in that area. If the stinging does not stop in a few seconds, the needle can be removed, and either a new needle can be placed there or the area can be left to rest. Sometimes, that is all that is needed for an area to begin to unblock itself. At worst, a small bruise may show up there the next day. When each treatment is complete, the needles are painlessly removed and thrown away. The needles are only used once.

Treating Symptoms With Tuí Na

My dear friend Karen Moore, a Licensed Acupuncturist and Traditional Chinese Medicine Practitioner in Texas, explained to me that although in China acupuncture is used with all ages (including infants), in this country it is rarely used with children younger than 8 years of age. The exception is when absolutely necessary, such as to get a high fever down. Instead, Traditional Chinese Medicine practitioners use pediatric tuí na and Chinese herbs (see Chapter 10) with very young children. Pediatric tuí na is a form of Chinese massage that is gentle and easy to do with children. It is suitable for children younger than 12 years of age, but is especially designed for children younger than five. For children five and older, pediatric tuí na methods, in combination with the adult tuí na methods or herbs, is more appropriate.

As with acupuncture, pediatric tuí na balances the flow of energy in the body. The practitioner will work with the body's meridians and certain points along these natural energy channels, depending on the symptoms. According to Fan Ya-li, author of *Chinese Pediatric Massage Therapy*, the manipulations are generally "persistent, forceful, even, and soft so as to be deep and thorough...they should not be superficial, alternatingly heavy or light, too rapid or too short of duration." Fan Ya-li also explains that there are nine basic Chinese pediatric tuí na manipulations, each with its own purpose. The specific treatment used will be selected by the clinician and based on your child's symptom profile.

Are Acupuncture and Tuí Na Safe?

In general, the ancient healing arts of acupuncture and pediatric tuí na are viewed as safe, time-tested methods of health care. For the Chinese, these therapies have been a standard part of the health care system for over 3000 years. They are used safely and successfully on a regular basis, beginning in infancy and proceeding through the life span. I imagine that if there were any severe adverse reactions to these methods, we would have heard about them by now.

Treatment with acupuncture is generally pain-free, or may involve very little pain if a certain point on the body is particularly blocked. In that case, the only risk is of having a tingly feeling or a small bruise where the needle was placed. There is no risk of disease from the treatment, because today, acupuncturists use sterile needles that are individually wrapped and thrown away after one use. In terms of side effects, most people do not experience any adverse reactions to the treatment. For all of my searching, the only negative response I found suggested that very, very rarely, someone may experience what is called a "needle shock" reaction, including lightheadedness, slight nausea, vomiting, or fainting. This reaction is easily reversed by removing the needles and having the patient lay in the recovery position. One acupuncturist I spoke to has not seen any adverse reactions from patients in her several years of practice.

Are Acupuncture and Tuí Na Effective?

The use of Traditional Chinese Medicine methods for dealing with symptoms of AD/HD in the US is increasing. Basically, the trained practitioner will find where the imbalances are and will design an individualized treatment plan to address them. Whether the practitioner uses acupuncture, pediatric tuí na, or Chinese herbs (discussed in Chapter 10) to treat a patient is based on each person's unique profile. An experienced acupuncturist will be sensitive to your child's needs, and will use the method that will work best for them.

Acupuncturist Karen Moore observed what she calls "remarkable changes" in children with the symptoms of AD/HD as a result of treatment with pediatric tuí na. Her consultations with other Traditional Chinese Medicine practitioners indicate that children diagnosed with AD/HD typically show clinical improvement from the treatments. In Moore's experience, factors such as the child's diet, nutrition, and environment play a large role in their symptoms and their recovery. This fits with the Chinese model of the body as an energy system. The food we eat feeds and nourishes the blood and fluids of the body, which in turn support the body's organs, Qi (life force energy), Jing (essence), and Shen (mental alertness). She recommends diet and nutritional changes for most of the children she works with, to help the systems of the body function freely and in harmony with each other.

My personal belief is that, as with other treatments, the effects of Traditional Chinese Medicine therapies will be different for each unique person depending on their histories, readiness, openness, health issues, how severe their symptoms are, and how well they follow up with their treatment plan. Having experienced acupuncture myself, I can speak to the value of these treatments in leaving you feeling calm, centered, open, more present, better able to focus, stronger, looser and as if "all is right with the world." I have used acupuncture to deal with many specific health concerns over the years, including migraine headaches, insomnia, allergies, flu symptoms and fevers, symptoms related to my monthly cycle, and spasms in my diaphragm. With a well-trained practitioner, Chinese Medicine therapies can provide a safe, gentle and effective way to strengthen the body as a whole system, and to deal with your child's specific health needs.

What To Consider With Traditional Chinese Medicine Therapies

Keep in mind that in this country, for children younger than eight years, pediatric tuí na is recommended rather than acupuncture. You should know, however, that as of the writing of this book, licensed acupuncturists were not allowed to practice pediatric tuí na in some states, unless they also had a massage license. For example, the medical board in Texas decided that pediatric tuí na is considered manipulation, so practitioners must have a massage license to use this technique (in addition to their license in Traditional Chinese Medicine). Children eight years or older have access to acupuncture, though, if they are open to it.

The number of sessions needed, the frequency of the sessions, the number of needles used, and the amount of time per session will depend on the practitioner and on your child's unique situation. Things like the child's diet, their environment, the severity of their symptoms, how long they have had the symptoms, and how well they follow their treatment plan will affect the course of treatment. Typically, for children experiencing symptoms of AD/HD, it is recommended that they commit to weekly treatments for at least nine weeks, and then have a re-evaluation. Cost per session varies, but in Central Texas, it generally ranges from $35 to $75. Insurance companies typically do not cover energy therapies such as acupuncture and pediatric tuí na.

Finding a Traditional Chinese Medicine Practitioner

Training to become a licensed acupuncturist is very rigid and specialized. Practitioners get a degree in Oriental Medicine, and must also pass a national licensing exam to become a Licensed Acupuncturist (LAC) or a Certified Master Acupuncturist (CMA). Practitioners may also be a Doctor of Oriental Medicine (OMD), or may be listed as practicing Traditional Chinese Medicine (TCM). This means that they have the necessary training in acupuncture, tuí na, and Chinese herbs (discussed in Chapter 10).

The best way to find the right person to work with you and your child using Traditional Chinese Medicine therapies is to get referrals from people you know and trust. Another way to find out who the practitioners are in your area is to look up a TCM school or school of acupuncture near you. They usually have lists of practitioners. You can also get on-line or contact a related organization, such as the American Acupuncture Council (1-800-838-0383; www.acupuncturecouncil.com) or the national licensing board, at www.NCCAOM.com.

Be sure to ask the practitioner you select as many questions as you need to for your comfort. Here are some things to check out:

1. Insist on a Licensed Acupuncturist with at least three years of independent practice experience. Find out:
   - what licensure they have (e.g., CMA, LAC, OMD, TCM)
   - who their licensing agent is (e.g., national and state boards);
   - how many years of experience they have; and
   - if they are a member of any state or national organizations (e.g., American Academy Of Medical Acupuncture).

2. Look for a practitioner who:
   - has experience working with children diagnosed as having AD/HD;
   - is licensed to use acupuncture, tuí na, and Chinese herbs.

3. Be sure you feel safe and comfortable with what the practitioner is doing for your child. If you do not feel comfortable with something they say or do, talk to them about it. Be willing to make a change if this does not work.

Links Between Sensory Input and AD/HD Symptoms

During the past few decades, professionals have looked at how children with symptoms of AD/HD process sensory input from the environment. It is possible that there is a link between challenges with children's sensory processing and symptoms of AD/HD. Some findings suggest that there is a type of sensory scrambling, overload or sensitivity that happens with at least some of these children, and that when this issue is addressed, their behavioral symptoms improve. In reviewing the research, there does appear to be a connection for some, but not all, children with symptoms of AD/HD. Let's take a closer look at this link.

Vision System Deficits

There is a new breed of optometrists calling themselves, "Behavioral" or "Developmental" optometrists that look specifically at how problems with the functioning of the visual system interfere with children's learning and behavior. These optometrists are not claiming that undetected eye problems are the cause of symptoms labeled as AD/HD, but they are suggesting that at least for some children, the behaviors can be the result of correctable deficits within the visual system. In these cases, a comprehensive vision exam, plus vision therapy, may be the answer. Optometrists maintain that the goal of a comprehensive vision exam is to rule out vision problems as the cause of children's challenging behaviors, which will minimize misdiagnosis as AD/HD or other disorders.

This is not a new idea. In fact, the assessment process for identifying *any* disability that may impact a student's learning requires that a vision screening be conducted to rule out visual deficits as the culprit. The problem is that the typical vision screening at school involves having students read a standard eye chart, which is not sufficient to detect the more serious visual deficits that these optometrists are talking about.

Dr. Judy Hughs, a full-service licensed Optometrist specializing in Vision Therapy at the Austin Eye Gym in Texas, explained that sight and vision are two different things. Whereas sight refers strictly to the ability to see, vision involves identifying, interpreting and understanding what you're seeing. A student can "see" with 2%20 vision, yet still be dealing with a weakness in some part of their visual system that keeps them from correctly interpreting and understanding what they see. These weaknesses can create behaviors that look like the ones we call AD/HD. Consider these facts:

1. The standard eye chart screening only catches 5% of vision problems.

2. How a child sees at 20/20 has nothing to do with how they see close up, which is needed for reading, writing, and drawing, for example.

3. Students can pass the standard eye chart, yet still have a serious vision deficit that goes undetected.

4. Special equipment and testing are needed to detect more serious vision deficits. Schools are not equipped to do this type of testing.

5. Deficits in any of the following aspects of vision can result in AD/HD-like behaviors:
   - eye teaming (binocularity vs. drifting);
   - laterality and directionality (left/right awareness);
   - visual tracking (moving the eyes from one point to another);
   - visual discrimination (telling one shape apart from another);
   - visual memory (the ability to remember what is seen);
   - visual motor integration (reproducing images through writing or drawing);
   - near- and farsightedness;
   - astigmatism (blurred vision); or
   - visual accommodation (the focusing system).

6. Serious vision deficits can lead to a number of behaviors that look like those we label as AD/HD. For example, the following DSM-IV criteria used to diagnose AD/HD can also be symptoms of a learning-related vision deficit:
   - does not attend to details; makes careless mistakes,
   - has trouble maintaining attention to tasks or activities,
   - does not seem to listen when spoken to directly,
   - has poor follow-through and low task completion,
   - has difficulty organizing tasks and activities,
   - avoids tasks requiring sustained attention,
   - often loses things,
   - is easily distracted,

- is forgetful,
- fidgets or squirms in seat,
- leaves seat without permission,
- talks excessively,
- blurts out answers out of turn,
- has difficulty waiting their turn,
- interrupts or intrudes on others

Serious deficits in the vision system can also result in behaviors such as clowning, work avoidance, resistance to visual tasks (such as reading, writing, drawing), and poor concentration. These behaviors may or may not be accompanied by the typical "red flags" of vision or reading difficulties, including losing their place while reading, using a finger or guide for tracking, jumbling words, having trouble copying, poor spelling and handwriting skills, letter or word reversals, misaligning words and numbers, headaches, rubbing their eyes frequently, experiencing eye strain, holding things close to their face, covering or closing an eye while working, and leaning or turning their head while working.

How Do You Test For a Vision Deficit?

To rule out a vision deficit, parents must take their children to an optometrist for a comprehensive vision exam. Special equipment is used to check the functions of the vision system and determine where the problem lies. The exam is not painful. The good news is that if a vision deficit *is* detected early, it can most likely be corrected through a program of vision therapy. An optometrist will determine whether the problem lies in the brain signaling system or in the eye response system. Then, through a series of exercises designed to teach, allow for practice, and provide feedback, either the brain can be retrained to provide the correct signals, or the eyes can be retrained to perform the brain signals correctly, or both, depending on the child's needs.

How Does Vision Therapy Work?

Dr. Hughes explained that typical vision therapy involves painless exercises done at the Optometrist's office and at home. A typical program can include anything from simple games, puzzles, and mazes used to strengthen the eye muscles, enhance eye-hand coordination and improve visual memory, to "sophisticated computerized optometric activities" used for training the eyes to work together, and to aid focusing, eye-aiming skills, and form perception skills.

Each therapy session is typically about 45 minutes long. Programs usually last from two to five months, but therapy can take as long as a year, depending on the severity of the deficit, the child's age, and the intensity of the program. The benefits tend to be long lasting since the therapy involves retraining the brain or parts of the vision system that are not working properly. Dr. Hughes suggested that behavioral and other improvements are usually seen by the eighth week of therapy.

What To Consider With Vision Therapy

Now that you know they exist, you can search for a Behavioral or Developmental Optometrist in your area. Check with anyone you know who may have a name to share with you, or look in the telephone book, make some calls, and ask some questions. Another option is to contact any of the organizations listed here for more information, or to ask for help finding the right person in your area for your needs:

1. College of Optometrists in Vision Development [www.covd.org]

2. Parenting: Pediatric Eye Care [www.children-special-needs.org]

3. The Stereo Vision Project [www.vision3d.com]

4. Parents Active for Vision Education (P.A.V.E.) [www.pave-eye.com]

5. American Optometric Association (AOA) [www.aoanet.org]

6. Optometric Extension Program (OEP) [www.oep.org]

7. Vision Help [www.visionhelp.com]

8. Optometrists Network [www.optometrists.org]

9. Attention Deficit Disorder [www.add-adhd.org]

Cost is something else that you will need to consider when selecting vision therapy for your child. A two-hour evaluation, plus a one-hour parent consultation, can range from $400 to $600. Therapy sessions can cost from $85 to $120 per session. Unfortunately, although most insurance companies will likely cover the cost of the evaluation, they generally do not cover the cost of the therapy. Keep in mind, however, that each insurance plan is different, so it is worth checking with your own insurance company.

Sensory Scrambling

Dr. Harold Levinson, a psychiatrist and neurologist, proposed the theory that some of the symptoms experienced by children diagnosed with AD/HD might be due to a problem in the inner ear, which regulates balance, voluntary movement, and energy levels. Dr. Levinson is the Clinical and Research Director at the Levinson Medical Center for Learning Disabilities. He has authored eight books and several scientific papers about cerebellar-vestibular (CV or inner ear) origins and treatments for dyslexia, learning disabilities, AD/HD, and anxiety or phobic disorders. He believes that inner ear problems cause "sensory scrambling" in the brain. This means that the brain cannot filter out distractions, which causes reading problems, symptoms linked to AD/HD, and other difficulties. It is true that many children diagnosed with AD/HD are often awkward, clumsy, poorly coordinated, and have a hard time with gross motor skills. Dr. Levinson suggests that anti-motion pills be used along with other drugs, including stimulants, to address the symptoms.

Dr. Levinson conducted controlled studies on four patients diagnosed with learning disabilities and CV dysfunction. He used anti-motion-sickness medications in different combinations with stimulant drugs (pemoline, methylphenidate, dextroamphetamine) to test for benefits. He concluded that combining the two types of drugs might have therapeutic value for treating children's symptoms, including those linked to AD/HD. These results, however, are premature and have not yet been validated through replication.

Although Dr. Levinson's clinical experience supports the inner ear theory, there is not enough scientific or clinical research to validate it or his claims about the usefulness of anti-motion pills for improving the symptoms linked to AD/HD. The usefulness of this treatment, as reported by testimonials from patients and his clinical experiences, however, is worth checking into. Inner ear problems have apparently been the culprit for at least a subgroup of people experiencing symptoms that are part of the AD/HD spectrum. Ruling out the possibility of an inner ear problem can be considered just as valid as ruling out a vision problem. Not every child diagnosed with AD/HD will have an inner ear problem, but some certainly may. Your child could be one of them. My feeling is that as with other treatment options, finding the best match for your child is a very individual process based on their unique situation.

Sensory Integration (SI)

A similar theory is based on the work of Dr. Jean Ayres, an occupational therapist. Her theory originated through her work with children diagnosed with autism and learning disabilities, and later, was expanded to included children with AD/HD, dyslexia, balance and coordination problems, sensory integration and motor skills difficulties, Asperger's Syndrome, Pervasive Developmental Disorders, and Down's Syndrome. Sensory integration is the ability to take in information from the outside world through the senses, and then organize, sort, interpret and connect it to something so that it makes sense in a way that allows you to respond. Dr. Ayres' theory says that if the brain cannot recognize and organize the information it receives through the senses, there is a problem with "sensory integration (SI)." Dr. Ayres believes that this is related to a dysfunctional vestibule (part of the inner ear). The vestibular system is linked to our ability to stay calm and alert. It works to balance the level of arousal in the central nervous system. When the vestibular system is not able to provide this balance, hyperactivity and distractibility can result.

Sensory integration problems can leave the brain either over- or under-stimulated, resulting in confusion, overwhelm, over-stimulation, withdrawal, and/or misperception of the world. A weakness in the SI system also leads to problems with balance, motor planning, attention, and perception. There may also be problems with learning, speech, coordination, behavior, and social skills. Since the input is also processed by the central nervous system, people with this weakness may be overly sensitive or easily overwhelmed by things, or feel "uncomfortable in their own skins." When there is disorganization in the central nervous system, developmental lags, and problems with behavior, emotions, and learning can result. The longer the problem continues, the more disorganized the input becomes, and the more confused the person feels.

Dr. Ayres created "sensory integration therapy" to deal with this weakness, which involves exercises designed to help the brain organize the information it receives. The Tomatis Method was also developed to stimulate the vestibular system. This method works with sound and sometimes movement to bring balance back to the functioning of the inner ear. The verdict is still out on this theory and these treatment techniques. My guess is that, as with other treatments, it will be successful for a subgroup of children with a certain profile of symptoms related to the diagnosis of AD/HD. In other words, it probably won't help everyone diagnosed with AD/HD, but it will likely help those with symptoms that may be related to an inner ear problem.

The Body-Brain Balancing Act

So you can see that as with other treatment options, balancing the functioning, structure, and/or energy of the body and brain can benefit some children with behavioral symptoms, yet is not a "magic bullet" approach for all children. I hope that you are beginning to understand that there is no "magic bullet" approach to children's symptoms, since each child is a one-of-a-kind Being in a distinct situation. This is why I believe that a holistic model is the most valid and safe way to approach their health. In my view, every child is worth the time and effort it takes to uncover their uniqueness and find the most useful solution for their symptoms.

10

NATURAL MEDICINE

Using homeopathy and herbs to stabilize children's moods and behavior

MANY PARENTS ASK me if natural medicines work, and if they are safe for themselves and for their children. People have heard the marketing and media information that, in my opinion, is generally not accurate. Parents have questions and are curious about the subject, but most do not have the time or energy to research it themselves. So, many have asked me about it.

I am not an expert in the area of natural medicine. It is simply a way of life for me – by choice. I began my journey into the natural medicine world over twenty-five years ago, after being disillusioned with the allopathic (or medical) model of prescribing drugs for my symptoms - drugs that did not always work, and that had worrisome side effects for my body. Today, I use natural, organic agents in every area of life, from my toiletries, to my cleaning products and laundry detergent, to my diet and health care, to my pet care. Just about everything you will find in my home is "green," meaning that it is earth friendly, organic and natural. I recycle glass, cardboard, paper, cans and plastic. And although I do my own research on natural health care and medicine products, I use a holistic doctor and dentist for their expertise. They know all the fine points that I may not have access to or experience with. Folks who know me know this, so they ask me questions about it.

Most of us have had very little exposure to natural medicines growing up; it was simply not the ruling way of life for the majority of

Americans in our generation. Luckily, there are still many folks that carry on the tradition of creating, studying, marketing, and using natural medicine products. This gives consumers like you and me a true choice when it comes to our health care. Like most people interested in a more natural way of life, I do believe that allopathic medicines and techniques have a place in our health care system. The allopathic or medical model simply does not provide me with a guide that I can live my life by. Holistic health, on the other hand, does. So, I live my life under the model of holistic health, and I rely on allopathic medicine for emergencies and critical care treatments.

So, people ask me, "Are natural medicines safe and do they work?" My answer to both of these questions is, "Yes, for me." What this means is that how a person responds to a natural agent (just as with conventional medicines) is a very individual experience because we are all unique. In general, though, there is not much mystery left to natural agents because they have been studied and used for centuries, much longer than conventional, man-made drugs. The people who work with them are medicinal experts. The information they collect is not only available to those who seek it, but it is valid and reliable. Each natural medicine has a specific action on the body that is known and understood by those who have spent their lives studying and using them. We also have enough information to know when precautions are in order and under what circumstances. I do recommend finding a holistic doctor to work with, because they are the experts in their field, just as allopathic doctors are.

Here is a list of who to look for when seeking a naturopathic doctor:

Doctors who are trained in natural medicine:
Naturopaths (N.D.)
Naturopathic Doctors (N.D.)
Naturopathic Physicians (N.D.)
Natural Medicine Doctors (N.D.)
Traditional Chinese Medicine Doctors (TCM)
Oriental Medicine Doctors (OMD)
Licensed or Certified Acupuncturists (L.A. or C.A.)
Homeopathic Physicians
Doctors of Homeopathy

Osteopathic Physicians (D.O.)
Herbalists
Certified Clinical Nutritionists (C.C.N.)
Other professionals who may have training in natural medicine:
Doctors of Chiropractic (D.C.)
Family Nurse Practitioners (F.N.P.)
Physician's Assistants (P.A.)

The Use of Natural Agents

There are many excellent sources of information out there about natural medicines that can be used to treat the symptoms we call AD/HD. I have summarized three of the more widely accepted ones in this section for you: homeopathy, herbs and Chinese herbs.

The information presented here is intended as a resource guide to help you with your search for natural agents in treating symptoms. *It is not meant to replace the advice of an expert. I recommend that you consult with a licensed naturopathic or holistic doctor before trying natural agents as treatment for specific symptoms.* This is because individual factors must be considered before a decision can be made about the usefulness and safety of any agent for a child. Just as you would not want to give your child the wrong type or dose of cough medicine, for example, you would not want to give them the wrong type or dose of a natural medicine.

May I remind you that all of us display the behaviors that we call AD/HD to some degree. They are a part of the normal range of behaviors that people are capable of. To be considered a "symptom", a behavior must be present to an *extreme* degree, meaning that it is much more frequent, intense, and/or long-lasting in your child than in the majority of other children of your child's age and level of functioning. True symptoms typically interfere with a child's ability to do the things that are a part of their average life, like get along with others, complete tasks, play, and respect boundaries.

So for example, difficulty sleeping once or twice a week is not extreme, especially for excitable children, and may not be considered a symptom. If a child has difficulty sleeping *every* night, however, and the lack of sleep is disrupting their ability to function during the day, that could be a symptom of something larger. As with most symptoms, difficulty sleeping can be caused by many things, such as nutritional issues, excitability, stress, lack of exercise, worry, nightmares, trauma, or fear. That is why it is important to work with a holistic doctor (e.g., a naturopath or homeopath) who can accurately assess your child's situation and provide a unique treatment program for their needs.

Keep in mind that the natural agents discussed in this section are not "magic bullets" meant for *curing* the symptoms linked to a diagnosis of AD/HD; no drugs or medicines are. The best approach is a holistic one that addresses the whole child. It is my opinion that natural medicines, just as pharmaceutical medicines, are best used as a compliment to other interventions discussed in the earlier sections of this book, such as parenting and behavior management strategies, lifestyle changes, or biophysical methods.

Having said that, natural medicines *are* an important part of holistic health care. Consider this example: A child is behaving in an overactive manner. Let us say that this over-activity is due to an allergy to wheat. Although natural agents may help to bring the child's body back into balance and calm the symptom of over-activity, it will continue to return until the wheat allergy is identified and managed through dietary changes. If the diet is not changed, every time the child eats a product containing wheat, the over-activity will resume. This will set up a cycle in which the balancing action of the natural agent is battling against the imbalancing action of the wheat, probably with little or inconsistent overall effects.

The same would be true if pharmaceutical drugs were used to soothe the symptoms without addressing the underlying cause. The drugs may temporarily calm the symptoms that children experience, but they do not provide a long-term cure. They may help the brain produce more neurotransmitters, for example, but they do not address the reason why neurotransmitter production is out of balance in the body in the first place.

The exception to this may be when there is an identified illness, brain injury or head trauma that resulted in a permanent physical shift in which the brain's ability to function normally has been compromised. Then, the illness, brain injury or head trauma becomes the underlying cause of the imbalance. In this case, either natural agents or pharmaceutical drugs may be needed on a permanent basis to persuade the brain to function as intended. Otherwise, I believe that natural agents and pharmaceutical drugs alone, although helpful for symptom management, may not address the underlying causes of the symptoms we call AD/HD.

For some, natural medicines provide a similar type of symptom relief that strong pharmaceutical drugs may provide. However, the actions of natural agents on the body are generally slower, more gentle, and more in sync with the body's natural healing abilities than pharmaceutical drugs. The natural agents essentially support the body in healing itself by helping to bring its systems into balance, and to do their jobs more efficiently and effectively. Because of their more subtle nature, they are not the best choice for critical times when symptoms are intense, severe or dangerous. For these times, the potency and fast-acting nature of pharmaceutical drugs may be a better choice, at least in the short term.

The Safety of Natural Medicines

It is important to be mindful that natural substances, just as pharmaceutical substances, have an effect on the body. The differences lie in their potency, their chemical makeup, and how they work with the body's natural systems. Before using *any* substance - natural or pharmaceutical - it is best to consult with a trained health care provider who can evaluate its usefulness in your situation. Too much or too little of *any* substance can create unwanted effects in the body. Allergic reactions or sensitivities, substance interactions, and possible adverse events (or side effects) are also concerns.

The reality is, though, that there are far fewer reports of such concerns with the use of natural medicines than there are with pharmaceutical drugs. We can still ask, however, whether this is due to the safety of natural medicines or to a lack of reporting. With all the tracking and recording of adverse reactions to pharmaceutical drugs, we are still only aware of between 1% and 10% of actual incidents. This means that there are likely many more adverse reactions and side effects to pharmaceutical drugs than physicians are aware of. Unlike pharmaceutical drugs, however, people have safely used the majority of natural medicines available today for health care for centuries. I would venture to guess that since their use is rapidly increasing in this country ($11 billion in sales a year and rising), we would have heard stories by now about life-threatening or fatal reactions. As it stands, I am aware of only three situations in which adverse reactions have resulted from the use of natural medicines:

- when too much of an herb was accidentally taken, causing toxicity in the body;

- when there was an allergic reaction to an herb; and

- when an herb was taken in combination with a pharmaceutical drug that had a similar action on the body (for example, taking St. John's Wort for depression while on a prescription antidepressant).

There are always professionals, such as doctors and psychiatrists, who consider what they call "alternative medicines" (referring to homeopathics and herbs) to be dangerous, particularly for children. They base their concerns on the fact that these medicines "are largely untested in children and may have serious health consequences." This view was expressed by physicians at the American Academy of Pediatrics' annual meeting in December 2001, in San Francisco. The physicians reported that about 20% of children appear to be using alternative medicine, and they are concerned about the lack of studies on how these medicines affect children.

I am surprised by this line of questioning, when for years, this same concern has been raised about pharmaceutical drugs by many medical and health professionals. The first study of the effects of stimulants on children younger than six years of age just began in 2002. Before this time, the drugs had *not* been tested for use with this age group. However, drugs for the symptoms of AD/HD, anxiety, and depression are frequently prescribed to children ages six and younger by physicians and psychiatrists anyway. These doctors choose to make guesses (albeit educated ones) about how much of a drug to give these youngsters, and what the effects should be, based on how they work with adults, even though the short- and long-term effects of the drugs on young children's development is unknown. Today, as the use of pharmaceutical drugs with children increases, reports are being made public of life-altering, life-threatening, and even fatal responses to some of them, such as Cylert and Adderall, as noted in Chapter 1. This has not been the case with natural medicines.

With this in mind, I present you with three natural options (or agents) that have clinical and/or scientific support for their effectiveness with the symptoms of AD/HD. In this chapter, you will read about homeopathy, general herbalism, and Chinese herbs. I review basic information about each one, what is known about their safety and effectiveness, how to choose and use them, what to avoid, and specifics about using them for symptoms of AD/HD. There are also many books and magazines available about these natural medicines. I encourage you to spend some time learning about one or more of them as generally more safe and gentle alternatives to pharmaceutical drugs for your child's health care.

Homeopathy

The simplest way to describe homeopathy is the principle that natural substances that can create symptoms if given to a healthy person, can relieve those same symptoms if given to a sick person. This principle is known as the "Law of Similars" and was popularized by a German physician and chemist who became fascinated with the idea and eventually created the first homeopathic medicines. His name was Samuel Hahnemann. He ran across the idea while translating ancient texts into German to support himself after becoming disenchanted with the medical practices of his day, and giving up his own medical practice. He encountered some writings of Hippocrates from around 400 B.C. which stated, "Through the like, disease is produced, and through the application of the like it is cured." Although Hippocrates, known as the "Father of Medicine," and Phillippus Paracelsus, a Swiss doctor and alchemist, had taught this practice in earlier times, it did not become popular until Dr. Hahnemann revived it. For this reason, Dr. Hahnemann is considered the founding father of homeopathy.

Dr. Hahnemann eventually developed and tested several homeopathic medicines, or "remedies," which were successfully tried during the cholera epidemics of the 1830s in Europe. Whereas his patient death rate was less than 20%, that of the other doctors was more than 50%.

Homeopathy was also successfully used to treat other epidemic diseases such as malaria, typhoid, yellow fever, and scarlet fever during the early 19th century. Closer to modern times in 1996, sales of homeopathic remedies in the U.S. were said to be growing by 20% each year. I imagine that this figure is even higher today. You could argue that if they didn't work or if they had negative effects, so many people wouldn't be continuing to buy them. Let's take a closer look.

Are Homeopathic Remedies Safe?

Homeopathic remedies have been around for centuries, if we begin counting with Dr. Hahnemann's work (even longer if we go back to the work of Hippocrates and Paracelsus). Today, the Food and Drug Administration recognizes and regulates homeopathic remedies as over-the-counter medicines. Also, homeopathic pharmacies must follow rigid guidelines kept by the Homeopathic Pharmacopoeia of the United States. Homeopathic remedies have no side effects, and are non-addictive. Generally, the only problem a person may experience while taking a remedy is an allergic reaction, which will go away when the remedy is stopped.

Boiron®, one of the leaders of homeopathy, describes the remedies as using micro-doses of natural substances that work by stimulating the body's own healing response. They provide the body with a tiny, gentle amount of a natural substance so that the body only gets the amount it needs to promote self-healing. The use of micro-doses guarantees no toxicity or side effects, which makes them safe for children and adults. Also, Boiron reports that homeopathic medicines can be used with pharmaceutical medicines without interference due to the use of the micro-doses.

Be aware that with homeopathic remedies, there may be a worsening of symptoms before they get better. This change could last from a few hours to more than a week. There are also certain things that should be avoided during treatment with homeopathic remedies because they interfere with the effects of the remedy on the body. Consult your naturopathic or homeopathic doctor for more information about this, but some of the more common things to avoid include coffee, eucalyptus, camphor, menthol, recreational drugs, alcohol, electric blankets, topical medications, oral antibiotics and cortisone products (except in emergencies), and possibly acupuncture.

Are Homeopathic Remedies Effective?

Peter Chappell, one of the founders of the Society of Homeopaths, who has taught homoeopathy for decades in the UK and in Europe, describes homeopathic remedies as "powerful, effective healing energies often derived from serious natural poisons but not given in a poisonous dose." Homeopathic remedies come from minerals, metals, plants, and animal and human disease products.

The medicinal effects of homeopathic remedies are based on two principles: the *Law of Similars* and *potentization*. The Law of Similars, as mentioned before, is the concept of "like cures like." Potentization is the strength of the remedy. The potentization of the medicine is created by repeating two processes many times: *dilution,* or mixing the herbs with a water and alcohol solution to remove toxicity, and *succussion,* in which the medicine is violently shaken to evenly distribute the liquid. Succussion allows the medicine to keep its ability to work after dilution and actually makes it stronger. Hahnemann discovered that the process of potentization (repeatedly diluting and shaking the remedies) resulted in a medicine that had no side effects, was easily made, and was a strong curative.

Reichenberg-Ullman and Ullman, authors of the book, *Ritalin Free Kids,* maintain that homeopathy has been widely accepted and used with significant clinical success for at least 200 years in many parts the world. They dispel the myth that says homeopathy works through a 'placebo effect' (meaning that they only work when a patient *believes* that they will work) by pointing out that:

1. homeopathic medicine does not always work on patients who believe that it will;

2. homeopathic medicine works on patients who believe that it won't;

3. patients may respond to one homeopathic medicine but not to another; and

4. homeopathic medicine works well on infants and animals.

Research addressing how well homeopathic remedies work for the symptoms of AD/HD is difficult to find because federal funding in this area has been scant. Hopefully this situation will shift in the future. However, clinical investigations done by doctors who use homeopathic remedies with their patients show that they are extremely safe, nontoxic, and effective for treating conditions unrelated to symptoms of AD/HD for all age groups. One research review of over 100 studies on the effectiveness of homeopathy found that in 76% of them, homeopathic treatments were successful. The studies included treatments for such issues as infections, digestive disorders, influenza, hay fever, rheumatoid arthritis, fibromyalgia, recovery from surgery, psychological problems, asthma and pediatric diarrhea.

Doctors who use homeopathic remedies define them as effective when a patient's symptoms are better by at least 50% within one month, with a lasting effect of at least one year. Many times, the symptoms are noticeably better within a few days or weeks, and usually by 70% or more. How long this relief lasts depends on such issues as the vitality of the patient, how severe the symptoms are, factors in the environment, stress, and exposure to influences that can interfere with treatment. With the symptoms of AD/HD, the benefits from one dose of a homeopathic remedy can last four to six months.

I have used natural healing, including homeopathic medicines, as my primary method of health care for my self and my pets for over 20 years now. I have successfully used homeopathic remedies for treating cold and flu symptoms, nausea, bone trauma, muscle/soft tissue injury and soreness, cuts, bruises, headaches, nosebleeds, allergies, digestive issues…the list goes on. My primary care physician of the past five years is a naturopathic doctor who has been able to get rid of many long-standing symptoms I'd had that allopathic doctors couldn't resolve without the use of prescription drugs or surgery.

What I appreciate the most about this work is that it is completely holistic, tending to my mental, emotional, physical and spiritual/energetic bodies so that I stay in healthy balance in all aspects of myself. This is what science is showing us today – that we are several bodies in one, and that true health means that all aspects of us are vital and functioning at their best levels. Being healthy means we have vibrancy in our thoughts, feelings, physical status, beliefs and energy.

In their book, *Ritalin Free Kids*, Reichenberg-Ullman and Ullman provide one of the best discussions about homeopathy and the treatment of AD/HD that I have found. I encourage you to review it for yourself, if you are interested in this topic. The information I review here on the benefits of using homeopathics, plus when they are not recommended, comes from their book.

Benefits of using homeopathic treatment for AD/HD
It focuses on the whole person. It gets to the root of the problem. It is considered to be safe and effective. It does not have the side effects of prescription medications. It uses natural, nontoxic medicines. It treats each person individually. It addresses physical, mental, and emotional symptoms. It lasts for months or years, whereas prescription medications only last for hours. It is inexpensive. It gives you a lot of benefit for a little money. It is compatible with other therapies (e.g., counseling, biofeedback, etc.)

There are some situations in which homeopathic treatment may not be the best choice. I have already mentioned one, and that is when a health issue is in a state of crisis. Here are four others discussed by Reichenberg-Ullman and Ullman:

1. When youngsters are determined to sabotage the treatment by not complying, refusing to go to appointments, refusing to take the medicines, or by using substances that interfere with the treatment, such as caffeine or recreational drugs.

2. When parents do not agree on the usefulness of homeopathy, or when they are not willing to try it for at least six months.

3. When the symptoms have expanded into severe behavioral problems requiring inpatient treatment (e.g., jail, rehabilitation center, treatment center) rather than outpatient treatment.

4. When parents are looking for a "quick fix;" homeopathic medicines are slow-acting, not fast-acting like strong prescription drugs. They require patience and persistence, but their effects are long lasting.

Taking Homeopathic Remedies

Homeopathic remedies are sold in most health food stores in bottles with labels that tell what they are for and how they are to be used. The remedies come in several different forms, including tiny pellets, tablets, liquids, suppositories, and ointments. The pellets, tablets, and liquids are taken under the tongue (sublingually) due to the large number of capillaries found there which quickly carry them to the bloodstream. Your homeopathic or naturopathic doctor will recommend the best choice and form to address your unique situation.

Homeopathic Remedies For The AD/HD Diagnosis

I recommend that you talk to your health care provider before using homeopathic remedies with your child. There is more to these remedies than I have included here. The examples I provide in this book are just that: *examples*. They are intended as a guide to give you a place to begin your search for alternatives to drugs. With the help of a naturopathic or homeopathic practitioner, you can select the remedy that will work best for your child's symptoms. I recommend that you consult a trained practitioner, however, since each child's situation is unique and will call for a unique remedy. As Reichenberg-Ullman and Ullman say:

> The challenge in homeopathy is to pick the one substance from nature that truly matches the patient's symptoms. Rather than giving many different drugs to a patient, a

homeopath gives only a single natural medicine that is individualized according to the patient's pattern of symptoms. Homeopaths treat the *patient* not the disease. This means that ten patients with ADD may need ten different homeopathic medicines. Their individual differences are what lead the homeopath to choose a particular medicine that can help each of them lead a happier, better adjusted, more productive life. The homeopathic medicine must match the patient's symptom pattern or picture in order to be effective. When the match is made well and the prescription is correct, the patient will markedly improve physically, mentally, and emotionally.[9]

I found several homeopathic remedies that address the symptoms of AD/HD. I provide some examples here for you to consider. The names may vary slightly, but anyone familiar with homeopathics can help you select the correct one:

Hyperactivity. Many children diagnosed with AD/HD are described as being overactive, impulsive, impatient, as rushing or "racing" all day, or as having racing thoughts. Although each child's situation is unique and will need to be assessed as such, there are several homeopathic remedies that address these specific symptoms. For example, *Nux Vomica* and *Sulphur* might be good choices. You might also check into *Ignatia, Medorrhinum, Silica,* or even *Argentum Nitrate.*

Inattention. For those children whose symptoms lean toward distractibility and inattention, there are homeopathic remedies that address being absorbed in thought and/or indecisive. For instance, *Pulsatilla* and *Sulphur* can be helpful for these symptoms. Also, *Natrum Mur* and *Nux Vomica* could be considered.

Insomnia. Sleeplessness is often a symptom for children diagnosed with AD/HD. Some children taking prescription stimulants for their hyperactivity are also given a prescription sedative to help them sleep at night. Dr. James Duke, who has a Doctorate Degree in Botany and spent 32 years studying medicinal plants and herbs for the U.S. Department of Agriculture, explains in his book, *The Green Pharmacy,* that although artificial sedatives work, "they can become addictive, and they interfere with natural sleep cycles." They can also leave you feeling groggy in the morning.

As an alternative, consider trying homeopathic remedies that can help children sleep at night in a gentle, non-invasive way. For example, these natural remedies are safe for children, non-addictive, do not interfere with natural sleep cycles, and do not leave you feeling "hung over" in the morning: *Kali Phosphoricum, Nux Vomica,* and *Ignatia.*

Homeopathic Formulas For The AD/HD Diagnosis

There are some companies that have created combination formulas of homeopathic remedies to address certain symptom profiles. For example, Boiron makes a few "homeopathic specialty products" that are designed to work on specific symptoms. Three that may be useful in dealing with symptoms associated with AD/HD include *Ginsenique,* for relieving fatigue; *Quietude,* for helping with sleep problems; and *Sedalia,* for calming stress. Consult with your doctor or contact Boiron for specific information about these formulas (1-800-264-7661).

Guidelines For Using Homeopathy

According to Reichenberg-Ullman and Ullman, the following guidelines can help you get the best results from using homeopathic treatments:

1. Find a well-trained homeopath that you trust.
2. Try it for six months to one year.
3. Be honest and thorough with your homeopath.
4. Tell your homeopath about any other medications the child takes.
5. Be certain that you know what to avoid during treatment.
6. Be sure to attend follow-up appointments and report any changes in the child's health.
7. Do not try to self-treat.

Guidelines For Selecting a Homeopathic Practitioner

I want to take a moment to emphasize the importance of working with a trained homeopath, rather than trying to self-diagnose and treat symptoms. As Reichenberg-Ullman and Ullman noted:

> "there are over 2000 homeopathic medicines. It takes years of homeopathic study and practice to make the fine distinctions about when to prescribe which medicine. Although homeopathic medicines do not have long lists of side effects like many conventional medicines, it is also possible to experience a reaction to the medicine. IN ANY CHRONIC CONDITION, WHETHER PHYSICAL, MENTAL, OR EMOTIONAL, DO NOT TREAT YOURSELF OR YOUR CHILD. Find an experienced homeopathic practitioner."[10]

A visit to a natural medicine doctor will save you much time and energy on trying to figure out what *might* work by yourself. These doctors can properly diagnose the symptoms and choose the best remedy for each individual. With their help, you can get right to the root of the problem and begin to address it immediately. For severe conditions, homeopathic and naturopathic doctors have access to special remedies that are more potent than those sold in stores. They also monitor progress, make changes as needed, and know how to handle an unexpected reaction to a treatment. Most are willing to consult with patients by phone when questions arise. The sense of safety and comfort that this type of relationship provides is well worth any investment you might make in terms of time or money.

Ideally, when selecting a natural medicine doctor to work with, you want to check if they:

1. practice classical homeopathy;
2. are board certified or very experienced;
3. spend at least an hour with new patients getting detailed information;
4. prescribe one homeopathic medicine at a time; and
5. wait at least 5 weeks before checking the patient's progress.

Herbs

The use of herbs for health and healing is not a new practice. Herbs and herbal medicines have been an integral part of life and health care across cultures throughout history, particularly with indigenous or native populations. It is only more recently (in this century), however, that they have begun to receive more attention by health care practitioners in the U.S. So, although herbal medicines may seem "new" to us in this country, they are in fact one of the oldest forms of medicine and are the foundation for many man-made medicines we use today.

The World Health Organization has been supportive of traditional, or herbal, medicines since 1977. Herbal medicine can include botanical herbs, flowers, seeds, bark, roots, and the heart wood of trees. David Hoffman, a leading expert in the field of herbal medicine, trained with the National Institute of Medical Herbalists, President of the American Herbalist Guild, Director of the California School of Herbal Studies and author of *The Herbal Handbook*, writes that what may not be known to the general public is that "herbs are the foundation of much of modern medicine. This is a result of many years of scientific research into the active ingredients of plant remedies." Some examples are aspirin, which comes from *Willow Bark*, and steroids, which come from *Wild Yam*. Actually, nature has been a part of our survival from the beginning of time. We humans successfully relied on nature to meet all of our needs at one time.

Herb Safety

Any substance, including herbs, can be harmful in the wrong amounts for a person's body, or in combination with certain factors or substances that don't work with each other. In general, though, herbal medicines are considered safer than conventional (or pharmaceutical) medicines because, as master herbalist Dr. James Duke explains, conventional drugs are in concentrated formulations to be fast-acting, which can result in more severe side effects. Herbal medicines are more dilute and tend to have fewer and less severe side effects than conventional medicines.

Although herbs are more dilute than conventional drugs, they are not as dilute as homeopathic medicines; they fall somewhere in between homeopathics and conventional drugs in terms of their strength. And, although herbal medicines are generally viewed as safe for adults and children, and side effects are rare, they are considered medicinal because they have a direct "action" on the body. Some individuals may have unknown sensitivities to certain herbs that could result in such things as rashes, headaches or nausea that disappear when they stop taking the herb. Still, side effects from herbs are generally less severe and easier to manage than those produced by pharmaceutical drugs.

Some Herb Cautions

According to Dr. Alan Agins, Pharmacologist and Adjunct Associate Professor at Brown University Medical School, there are five herbs that may be dangerous in certain situations. These include:

1. Comfrey - for swelling around broken bones. When taken internally, it can disrupt blood flow to the liver and may cause liver failure.

2. Ephedra (Ma Huang) - for bronchial congestion and asthma symptoms. As a stimulant, it may increase heart rate and blood pressure. It should be avoided by those with diabetes, high blood pressure, heart problems, and thyroid abnormalities. In large doses, it can cause dizziness, insomnia, and vomiting.

3. Homegrown Mint - for upset stomach. Spearmint and Peppermint are safe, but Pennyroyal mint plants have a poisonous oil that can cause liver failure or death if ingested. It is hard to tell the plants apart.

4. Senna, Cascara Sagrada, Buckthorn Bark - for constipation. If taken for a long period of time, they can cause diarrhea, which can result in electrolyte imbalances that can create heart problems.

5.   Willow Bark - for relieving pain and reducing fever. This herb contains low amounts of salicin, the active ingredient in aspirin. It can cause stomach irritation and Reye's syndrome in children. Reye's syndrome is a brain disease involving fever, vomiting, fatty infiltration of the liver, and swelling of the kidneys and brain.

I recommend that you consult a trained herbalist or naturopathic doctor if you are interested in treating symptoms with herbs. Working with an herbalist saves you time and energy spent on the "guesswork" about what may be causing the symptoms, and on what the best treatment approach will be. They can also identify what to do if there are unexpected reactions to an herb or interactions between the herb and other substances. These experts can provide treatment safety for you and your child by:

- accurately diagnosing the problem;
- providing you with an individualized treatment plan based on the uniqueness of the symptoms and situation;
- monitoring herb combinations;
- monitoring and managing drug, herb, and food interactions;
- monitoring allergic reactions; and
- providing clear information about what to expect and what should be avoided while taking an herb.

Are Herbal Medicines Effective?

Herbal agents are considered medicinal because they have an affect on the systems of the body. They help the body heal itself. They can, for example, balance body chemistry, strengthen the immune system, fight infections, soothe sore or inflamed muscles, calm the emotions, and help ease sleep and digestive difficulties. As natural medicines, herbs are gentle and slow-acting on the body, compared to pharmaceutical medications, which are powerful and fast-acting. Oftentimes, there must be a build-up of herbal medicine in the body before symptoms begin to disappear.

How long it takes for an herb to have an affect on the body depends on the herb itself. Some are stronger than others and take less time, while the more gentle herbs will take more time. Basically, herbs work on the body in one of three ways:

1. as "**Challengers**," which trigger a protective response within the body;

2. as "**Normalizers**," which persuade the organs and tissues to return to normal functioning; and

3. as "**Eliminators**," which support the eliminatory organs in doing their job, including the bowels, kidneys, skin and lungs.

There is little research comparing herbal treatments to pharmaceutical drug treatments, yet Dr. Duke reports that oftentimes, herbs have successfully treated "conditions that high-tech pharmaceuticals could not touch." Many herbs have also been found to work as well as, or in some cased better than, their pharmaceutical counterparts. For example, Ginger has been shown to work better than dimenhydrinate (Dramamine) for motion sickness. St. John's Wort is another one: it has repeatedly performed equal to, or better then, pharmaceutical antidepressants for mild forms of depression.

Research *has* been done that compares the effectiveness of herbs with a placebo (a "blank" pill with no action on the body). In this type of research, a placebo is given randomly to certain subjects, while other subjects are given the herb being studied. Subjects are not told which one they are taking. Researchers then determine the herb's effectiveness compared to the placebo. In this type of research, herbs have generally had either a positive effect on symptoms, or no "significant" effect, when compared to a placebo. I have not reviewed reports of negative responses to herbal treatments.

Using Herbs

When taking herbal agents, consult with an herbalist or naturopathic doctor, or follow the instructions on the label, to determine the correct dosage for your specific situation. Ed Smith, an expert herbalist, and internationally known teacher and lecturer on herbs and herbal healthcare for more than 20 years, suggests using Clark's Rule to convert adult dosages to a child's dose. The Rule says to "divide the child's weight (in pounds) by 150 to get the approximate fraction of the adult dose to give to the child." For example, a 50-pound child would get $5\%_{150}$ (or $\frac{1}{3}$) of the adult dose. So, instead of 30 drops, three times a day, the child would get 10 drops, three times a day.

Types of Herbal Medicines

You can find herbal preparations in many forms, including tonics or teas, tinctures or liquid extracts, oils, pills or capsules:

Tonics are infusions in which boiling water is poured directly onto the dried herb, or plant leaf, to make a tea. You drink the tea according to the directions or to the instructions of your health care provider.

Tinctures are a concentrated liquid form of the herb that is extracted from the plant and dissolved in an alcohol and water mixture. These are also called "liquid herbal extracts." They are taken directly on the tongue or in a glass of cool or warm water. An example of a tincture used in baking is Vanilla extract. The alcohol in the tincture serves three purposes: it extracts and preserves the active components of the herb; it is a natural preservative; and it helps with absorption into the bloodstream.

Oils are also extracted from the plant and most are for external use only. They can be used in many forms, including as a massage agent, bath scent, body fragrance, body mist, toilet water, or inhalant. They can also be diffused or used in a vaporizer. See the discussion of aromatherapy with essential oils in Chapter 11, beginning on page 250.

Pills and capsules are a more processed form of the herb that can be taken like any other supplement, as described on the label or by a licensed practitioner. They are what is called "standardized," meaning that they contain a certain minimum amount of the main active ingredients of the herb.

Treating Specific Symptoms With Herbs

Herb expert David Hoffmann cautions against claiming that an herb will have a certain effect since herbal actions in the body depend on a person's special body chemistry and lifestyle. What may work for one person might not work for another person with the same symptoms. This is why it is important to consult an herbalist or naturopathic doctor who can work with a person's unique symptoms, check progress, and make changes as needed for relief. In reality, the same caution holds true for pharmaceutical drugs. Of course, the most powerful approach you can choose for your child will be based on the widest range of information and the broadest selection of "tools" that you have at your disposal. Herbal medicines are one more tool that you can place into your toolbox of possibilities.

In terms of treating the symptoms we call AD/HD, the effectiveness of herbs is unclear. Although herbal agents can help relieve some of the symptoms, they are not a "cure all" or a "magic bullet." They are not likely to get rid of the root cause of the behavioral symptoms your child is showing. Just as with homeopathic remedies, they will work best as a compliment to other treatment approaches which support the systems of the body in operating at optimum levels (or 100%), such as changes in nutrition and overall health care. They *can* provide a more gentle way to help calm symptoms than prescription drugs, because any side effects a child might experience will be very rare and minor.

Since the nervous system regulates both our physical and psychological wellbeing, it is to this system that we look for guidance in dealing with symptoms associated with a diagnosis of AD/HD. Research shows that *all* of our psychological processes are linked to the central nervous system, including our behaviors and emotions. The brain and the central nervous system work together to govern the body. You can make a positive difference in your child's functioning, then, by keeping their nervous systems healthy.

There is a certain class of herbs that helps to balance the nervous system in some way to create helpful change. These herbs are called "nervines" and include tonics, stimulants, and relaxants. Nervine tonics strengthen and restore the tissues directly. Nervine stimulants stimulate the overall functioning of the nervous system, and nervine relaxants calm and soothe the nervous system. The type of nervine that might be most helpful in your child's situation depends on what their profile is. Let's look at some nervine relaxants that are worth checking into for addressing symptoms linked to AD/HD.

Hyperactivity and restlessness. Many children with excessive energy have difficulty calming down in the evening to prepare for sleep, or have trouble falling or staying asleep. The following herbs are mild sedatives and relaxants that can be used to help with symptoms of restlessness, over-excitability, nervousness, sleeplessness, and anxiety. There are many others, but these are the ones that seem to have a fairly strong reputation among herbalists:

California Poppy – This herb is a non-addictive sedative that can help with over-excitability and sleeplessness.

Camomile or Chamomile – There are two kinds of Camomile, Garden and German varieties. Both are considered good, gentle sedatives for children. Camomile tea is readily available in stores.

Lemon Balm – This herb is also called "Melissa" or "Balm." It is known for its anti-depressive properties, as it can relieve stress, anxiety and tension.

Pasque Flower – This herb has a reputation for being a good relaxant and helps with nervous tension, insomnia, and general over-activity.

Passion Flower – Although this herb is widely used as a sedative in Britain and Germany, it is not yet readily available in over-the-counter preparations in the US. It is viewed by some herbalists as the herb of choice for dealing with chronic or stubborn insomnia. It does not leave you feeling "hung over" in the morning.

Skullcap – This herb has sedative and tranquilizing properties that can reduce nervous tension, restlessness, and irritability. It also restores the central nervous system.

Valerian - Although this herb has proven in research to be a very effective sleep aid, it is not considered habit-forming (like unnatural sedatives) and will not leave you feeling "hung over." It can help relieve tension, anxiety, and over-excitability.

Valerian-Passionflower Compound – This combination of herbs has a gentle sedative effect that soothes and quiets the nervous system.

Wild Lettuce – This herb is known for its ability to help with insomnia, restlessness, and excitability in children. It calms an over-active nervous system. It can be safely combined with Passion Flower or Valerian.

Inattention. For those children who tend to be distractible, inattentive, and day-dreamy, the following herbs have a strong reputation among herbalists as supporting mental functions:

Ginkgo or Ginkgo Biloba – This herb has the reputation of helping with alertness, memory loss, poor concentration, and poor mental performance by increasing circulation to the brain.

Gotu Kola-Ginkgo Compound – This combination is recommended for enhancing mental functioning by rejuvenating the brain and central nervous system.

Some parents have been led to believe that giving their children stimulants found in foods such as coffee, soda, or chocolate will calm them down. Keep in mind that stimulants like sugar and caffeine, which are highly accepted and used in our society, are hard on the nervous system. The shift in energy that they create is short-lived, leads to a "rollercoaster" effect on mood (extreme ups and downs), results in a worsening of symptoms once the effects wear off, and actually drains the body of needed nutrients. Using them as a "quick fix" to try to calm or boost your child's mood will leave them feeling worse than before in an hour or so.

Herbal Formulas For Symptoms of AD/HD

There are three herbal formulas for calming the symptoms of AD/HD that have been recommended by some experts in the field. The herbs in these formulations have specific actions in the body. This is why I encourage you to consult your naturopathic doctor or herbalist before using any of these formulas to get the best and safest match for your child's needs. The best way to obtain the formulas is through consultation with your naturopath. The formulas are:

Focus Formula - contains Oats, Lemon Balm, Hawthorne, Ginkgo, and Scullcap. These herbs also affect the central nervous system by calming the nerves and supporting the body's overall ability to deal with stress. Note that Hawthorne is a powerful herb that supports heart functioning and is used in treating heart problems.

Liquid Serenity - contains St. John's Wort, Kava Kava, Oats, Siberian Ginseng, Skullcap, Chamomile, Schisandra, and the essential oils of Lavender and Orange. These are all substances that influence the central nervous system and have tranquilizing properties. They address stress, depression, anxiety, nervousness, debility, or sleep problems. Kava Kava relaxes muscles. Schisandra supports the liver's ability to cleanse the body of toxins.

Melissa Supreme (or Compounded Melissa) - contains Lemon Balm, Chamomile Flowers, Passionflower, Skullcap, Wild Oat Seed, Gotu Kola, and Mineral Salts. These herbs also support the functioning of the central nervous system. They have relaxing properties to help with relieving stress, anxiety, and sleep problems.

What To Consider When Using Herbs

If you make the decision to treat your child's symptoms with herbal preparations, there are several guidelines that can make your journey easier. Here are some final points to think about before you begin.

Self-diagnosis. I discourage self-diagnosis. You want to be certain that you are on the right track with what you put into your child's body, herbal or otherwise. The easiest way to get onto the right track is to work with an herbal practitioner who already knows all of the "ins and outs" of treating symptoms with herbs. This is "the path of least resistance," so to speak. You can try to do it yourself, but it can be a fairly complex process. If you want to save some money, time and effort, work with a naturopath.

Communicating with practitioners. Be sure to tell your allopathic doctor (for example, your child's pediatrician) and your natural medicine doctor (for example, a homeopath or naturopath) about all the medicines your child is taking, including herbs. This practice will help you avoid unwanted medicinal interactions. If your child does have an undesired reaction, practitioners can determine the cause more easily when they know exactly what the child is taking. There are also herbs that have known effects on the body that may be unwanted in certain situations.

Buying herbal products. Today, herbal products are fairly popular, so most stores carry a wide selection. Standardized herbal products, such as those found on store shelves, have been processed more than bulk (loose, dried) herbs, which are usually found in containers, and measured and sold by weight. As noted above, the preparation of standardized herbs is regulated to guarantee a certain minimum amount of the main active ingredients. This is not so with bulk herbs; there is no way to know exactly how much of the active ingredients you are getting when you buy in bulk and prepare them yourself. Although standardized herbs are more expensive than bulk herbs, they are still significantly less expensive than their pharmaceutical counterparts. They are also easier to use because they save you planning and preparation time. The problem with standardized herbal products, though, is that they gradually lose potency when stored.

You may notice when you read the labels on standardized herbal products that they do not list claims of medicinal or therapeutic use - what the product is used for, what symptoms it treats, or possible side effects. This is due to the fact that the Food and Drug Administration requires a product to be approved as a "drug" before claims can be made about its safety or effectiveness, including possible side effects. Unfortunately, this process costs in the neighborhood of $200 million. Large pharmaceutical companies can afford this, and it is worth it to them, because they can patent their manufactured drugs. Patenting insures that they will make their money back from the sales of the drug. Not so with herbs, though, because you cannot patent a plant. And, as Dr. Duke said, "who in their right mind would spend millions to prove the benefits of a plant no one can patent?"

The results of this situation, however, are two-fold. First, since herbs cannot be patented, Dr. Duke explains that drug companies "make their money by pulling the medicinally active molecules out of herbs and then tinkering with them a little until they're chemically unique. The companies can then patent their new molecules, give them a brand name and sell them back to us for a lot more money than their original herbal sources cost."[11] Second, herbal products end up being sold without clear labeling, and consumers must buy the products without sufficient information - unless they work with a naturopath, homeopath, or other herbal expert, or take the time to educate themselves in a class, at the library, or in a bookstore.

Chinese Herbs

Chinese herbs have been a major part of the health care and healing system in China since at least 2000 B.C., although the first recorded list of herbs and their uses did not emerge until around A.D. 659. At the root of this system is the concept of harmony - supporting harmony among the systems of the body, and in harmony with the systems of nature. In this way, much of the focus of Chinese health care is on prevention through living a life that is in harmony with nature, and that supports the functioning of the body as a whole. As Dr. David Hoffman explains, nature is the guiding philosophical and spiritual principle and source of life to the Chinese. It is a way of being; it is "Dao" or "Tao," which means "the way."

Another concept at the root of Chinese medicine is that everything is made up of a balance of two forms (or sides) of the energy that is life: the dark ('yin') and the light ('yang'). Each side is associated with its own characteristics. For example, yin energy is considered cold, passive, and inactive; yang energy is considered warm, active, and full of movement. The Chinese believe that yin and yang *always* exist in balance of one another. When they are in balance in a person, the person is considered healthy. When they are out of balance, the person is considered to be in a state of disharmony and dis-ease. When working with a patient, Chinese doctors use certain methods to determine the source of their disharmony, and then choose herbs that specifically target different aspects of that disharmony.

Chinese herbs are viewed in terms of several qualities that relate to their actions in and on the body. These are:

- their perceived temperature, whether they are warm, hot, cool, cold, or neutral;

- their taste, whether they are pungent/acrid, sour/astringent, sweet, bitter, salty, or bland/neutral;

- their movement, whether they go upward and outward, or downward and inward; and

- what energetic channel, or meridian, an herb enters and targets.

So, a Chinese herbalist must consider how these qualities of an herb interact with each other to understand its function and action on the body. A Chinese herbalist must be able to select and/or prepare the herbs that will bring a patient's state of disharmony back into harmony, based on the best match between the symptoms and the qualities of an herb.

As with American herbs, Chinese herbal products come in several forms, including raw herbs, powdered herbs, tinctures, or as patent herbs (formulas that are manufactured). Patent herbs come in the form of pills or capsules, or as rubs, creams, sprays, and poultices for external use. Now, not only are many classic formulae imported from China, but there are manufacturers in the US who are creating their own variations of these products. This makes them easier to find, although I would still recommend working with an experienced Chinese herbalist before trying any of the products.

Are Chinese Herbs Safe?

Chinese herbology has been practiced in China since at least 2000 B.C. They have been used and passed down generation after generation, and are known to be safe. Additionally, all Chinese herbal products imported into the US must be approved by the Food and Drug Administration. They must be labeled as to the percentage of each individual herb in a formula, so practitioners know how much of the active ingredients are in a product. They must also carry a guarantee that they contain no metals. If an herbal product contains any metals that could be toxic, they are not allowed to come into this country. In addition, some Chinese herb companies have their own standards.

The Traditional Chinese Medicine practitioners that I consulted with had never experienced any adverse reactions to Chinese herbs with the children or adults they treated. The possibility exists, however, that someone may have an unwanted reaction to an herb, just as they might to any substance taken into the body. With Chinese herbs, it is possible that a child may get an upset stomach or have an allergic reaction, for example, to an herb or herbal formula. These reactions will go away when the formula is modified or stopped altogether. I don't know of any serious or fatal reactions to the use of Chinese herbal products, although *any* product, if misused, can create an adverse reaction in the body.

Are Chinese Herbs Effective?

The effectiveness of Chinese herbs, just as with other substances, depends on several factors. Historically, though, they have been used with safety and success to treat a variety of symptoms and conditions (both chronic and acute) for thousands of years. Because of the complex system of herbology used by the Chinese, it is important to work with a practitioner who is experienced with both the philosophy and the science of it.

Chinese Herbs For The Symptoms Of AD/HD

There is at least one Chinese herbal formula recommended by Master Chinese Herbalists for calming the symptoms of AD/HD. It is known as *Calm Dragon Formula*. Practitioners like it because it calms the energy without the side effects of pharmaceutical stimulants (e.g., it does not make you feel groggy or sleepy, and it does not create a cycle of emotional ups and downs). The others I read about are not easy to get a hold of, but have been shown in research to calm symptoms linked to AD/HD. These include Tiaoshen Liquor, Yizhi, and a combination containing Bupleurum Chinense, Scutellaria Baicalensis, Astragalus Membranaceus, Codonopsis Pilosula, Ligustrum Lucidum, Lophatherum Gracile and Thread of Ivory. If you are interested, consult with a Traditional Chinese Medicine practitioner to get more information about these formulas, and their usefulness in treating your child's specific symptoms.

Guidelines For Selecting An Herbal Practitioner

As with homeopathics, it is easiest and safest when working with herbs and Chinese herbs to consult a licensed practitioner who takes the "guess work" out for you. They are experienced and have access to products that you may not. They can do a thorough exam and determine the best approach for your child's unique lifestyle and profile of symptoms. Their expertise also makes it more likely that you will find something to help the situation more quickly.

When choosing a practitioner who works with herbs or Chinese herbs, consider:

1. getting a referral from someone you know;

2. their licensing and years of experience; look for Traditional Chinese Medicine Doctors (T.C.M.), Oriental Medicine Doctors (O.M.D.), Herbalists, Naturopaths or Natural Medicine Doctors (N.D.)

3. their experience with children and AD/HD-like symptoms;

4. how much time they spend doing an exam or an evaluation of your child's unique situation;

5. their willingness to answer your questions;

6. how comfortable you and your child feel with them.

Choose your naturopathic doctors just as carefully as you do your pediatrician or dentist. They can be a strong ally in dealing with your child's symptoms and keeping them in a balanced state of health and vitality.

11

AROMATHERAPY OILS AND FLOWER ESSENCES

*Gently encouraging the body to heal
and harmonize itself*

MOST PEOPLE HAVE probably heard of aromatherapy, but I suspect that only "alternative" types are familiar with flower remedies. Both are tools that focus on reaching the bodies deep, internal memories and patterns to create emotional and behavioral shifts. Both have some research behind them and fairly long histories of safe and effective use.

I have studied and used plant oils and flower essence remedies for years, and have spoken to numerous experts who deal with them at conferences and expos. I chose to include each of them in this book because I have found them to be effective at supporting folks in shifting subtle energetic and emotional patterns and blocks, which then leads to important shifts in behaviors. I am convinced that they offer something positive to the overall healing process. I also chose to include them in this book because I believe that it is important for you to have accurate and comprehensive information about as many options as possible for your child's situation. The more information you have, the better position you will be in to make up your own mind about what might be the best ones to try with your child. So, let's take a closer look at using aromatherapy and flower essences to shift behaviors.

Aromatherapy With Essential Plant Oils

Historical Uses Of Essential Plant Oils

People have known about the healing properties of essential oils for centuries. For instance, the Egyptians are credited as the first people to use oils as medicine. An ancient Egyptian "medicinal scroll", called the Ebers Papyrus, documents over 800 herbal prescriptions and remedies. It is believed to date back to 1500 B.C. They also used oils in ceremonies, rituals, and to open their minds for communicating with the spirit world. Recorded on the walls of the healing chambers in certain Egyptian temples are the names of oils they used to clear specific emotions. Egyptian King Tutankhamen's tomb contained around 50 alabaster jars holding oils. Egyptians and Babylonians used oils medicinally, to purify the air, and to protect against evil spirits. Mesopotamians, Romans, Indians, Aragians, Chinese, and Greeks also used oils for their healing properties.

There are 188 Biblical references discussing the use of oils, such as Frankincense, Myrrh, Rosemary, Hyssop, and Spikenard, for healing and protection from sickness. After the fall of the Roman Empire, the use of aromatherapy seems to have disappeared until the end of the 10th century when it reappeared in the Arab countries. It flourished for a time, and then disappeared again during the warring invasions of Mongolia and Turkey. Then it reappeared in Germany and among the Swiss around the 16th century. From that time on, it was used as the main source of healing until the rise of chemically produced medicines. Unfortunately, a great deal of knowledge about the benefits of essential oils was lost during the Dark Ages and during library burnings of old.

Modern Day Uses Of The Oils

In 1907, French Cosmetic Chemist, Dr. Rene'-Maurice Gattefosse', became interested in the healing properties of essential oils. He wrote a book about them that was published in 1937, called, "Aromatherapy." For this, he is considered the father of modern aromatherapy. He shared his research with a friend and medical doctor in Paris, Dr. Jean Valnet. Dr. Valnet successfully used therapeutic-grade essential oils when he ran out of antibiotics while treating injured patients in China during World War II. He is considered the first doctor to describe the use of essential oils for medical purposes. Dr. Paul Belaiche and Dr. Jean Claude Lapraz, two of Dr. Valnet's students, continued and expanded his research with the oils. They discovered that essential oils have antiviral, antibacterial, antifungal, and antiseptic properties, and that they oxygenate and carry nutrients into the cells.

Today, aromatherapy is seen as an important form of healing in Great Britain, France and Italy, and is beginning to get renewed support around the world and in the United States. In fact, medical training in France and England includes aromatherapy with essential oils, and if you travel there, you will find that many doctors in the hospitals use the oils. Only with the shift in our society toward homeopathic health care has aromatherapy with essential oils begun to gain recognition as an important healing tool in the U.S.

How Aromatherapy Works

Aromatherapy is the use of essential plant oils to encourage the body to tap into its self-healing powers. Essential oils are called "the soul of the plant" and are thought to awaken and strengthen the body's natural healing systems. The oils work holistically to balance the connection among the systems of our mind, emotions, body and spirit. Research also shows that aromatherapy with essential oils has cleansing and healing properties on the body. For example, the oils increase oxygen to the cells and directly affect the brain and other organs, our senses, and our mental and emotional states.

Essential oils are highly concentrated and so are much more potent than natural herbs, yet rarely have the unpleasant side effects that prescription or synthetic drugs create. When using pure, high-quality essential oils, they have antiseptic, antiviral, antibacterial, antifungal, antiparasitic, antimicrobial, anti-infectious, and hormone-balancing properties that stimulate and strengthen the body's immune system to help it stay healthy and free from illness. The oils also act as a delivery system to take nutrients directly to the cells. They are absorbed and assimilated into the body rather quickly (generally in 25 minutes or less), and do not leave any toxins behind. In fact, according to the *Essential Oils Desk Reference,* the oils "may detoxify the cells and blood in the body." When used in a diffuser, essential oils also change the molecular structure of the air by increasing the negative ions, which creates a clean, pure and refreshing air (ozone), rather then simply masking a bad odor.

D. Gary Young is a Doctor of Naturopathy (N.D.) with a Master's degree in Nutrition. Since 1985, he has traveled the world studying and researching the preventive, curative, and medicinal properties of essential oils, both from ancient and modern sources. His extensive investigation culminated in the creation of "Young Living Essential Oils" in 1989. Today, Young Living Essential Oils cultivates nearly 2000 acres of organic herb farmland in Idaho and Utah, and is one of the largest distilleries for organic therapeutic-grade essential oils in North America. Dr. Young is considered an expert and an authority on the subject of organic farming and germination, and therapeutic-grade essential oils.

In his book, *An Introduction to Young Living Essential Oils,* Dr. Young defines "frequency" as "a measurable rate of electrical energy flow that is constant between any two points. Everything has an electrical frequency, including essential oils." He explains the role of frequency in health and disease:

> "A healthy human body typically has a frequency ranging from 62 to 78 MHz (megahertz). Disease begins when the body frequency drops to 58 MHz. Clinical research shows that essential oils have the highest frequency of any natural substance known, creating an environment in which microbes cannot live."

According to the *Essential Oils Desk Reference,* since "essential oils are composites of hundreds of different chemicals, they can exert many different effects on the body." They also have chemical properties that make it difficult for bacteria to survive or spread. For instance, certain oils contain:

- aldehydes, which are antimicrobial and calming;
- eugenol, which is antiseptic and stimulating;
- ketones, which stimulate cell growth and liquefy mucus;
- sesquiterpenes, which soothe irritated tissue and affect emotions and hormonal balance; and
- phenols, which are strong antimicrobials.

The chemical structure of essential oils is "similar to that found in human cells and tissues," which makes them "compatible with human protein and enables them to be readily identified and accepted by the body." Like our own blood, they "fight infection, contain hormone-like compounds, and initiate regeneration."

Carolyn Mein, Doctor of Chiropractic, Acupuncture, and Bio-Nutrition, author, lecturer, and nutritional researcher, is a Fellow of the American Council of Applied Clinical Nutrition (F.A.C.A.C.N.), and a charter member and diplomat of the International College of Applied Kinesiology. In her book, *Releasing Emotional Patterns With Essential Oils*, she explains that

> "emotions have been found to be encoded within the DNA of the cells and passed on from generation to generation. Emotional behavior patterns have even been found to be 'locked' within families... Emotions themselves are stored in the body in its organs, glands, and systems. Since each organ has a vibrational frequency (or energy), as do emotions, the emotions will settle in an area with a corresponding frequency (e.g., anger is stored in the liver). Disease occurs when the body's vibrational frequency drops below a certain point. Essential oils can raise the body's frequency, and therapeutic grade (medicinal quality) oils are able to do this because they vibrate at a high frequency and transfer that frequency to the body."[12]

For all of these reasons, essential oils can play an important role in supporting the body's natural capacity to heal physically, as well as to stay healthy and balanced emotionally.

Are The Plant Oils Safe?

Essential oils are considered safe when they are pure (not diluted with anything synthetic), high quality, and when they are used properly. Standards for oil purity and quality were carefully and scientifically developed in Europe and are known as AFNOR (Association French Normalization Organization Regulation) and ISO (International Standards Organization). Buyers use these guidelines to separate therapeutic-grade essential oils from those that are of lower quality. *The therapeutic effects discussed in this book are only obtainable when using essential oils that meet the AFNOR and/or ISO standards.*

Always use oils as prescribed or as specified on the label. More is not necessarily better. In fact, using too much can be toxic. Generally, 60 drops of oil equals one teaspoon. If used incorrectly, certain oils can irritate the soft tissues of the body and disturb organ functioning. Keep in mind that the sense of smell in babies and children is much more sensitive than that of adults. For youngsters, an indirect application may be enough.

Some oils are more powerful than others, so it is helpful to have a guide to go by when using them. For example, tea tree oil is strong and can cause skin irritation if used repeatedly on the same spot in concentrated form. You can dilute the oils with any type of mixing oil, such as massage or pure vegetable oil. This can be helpful if a skin irritation develops after use. It is important to be aware and careful when applying oils to skin that may already have other personal care products on it such as make-up, soaps, lotions, and washes, especially those containing synthetic chemicals, ammonium, or petroleum- or hydrocarbon-based chemicals. These products can soak in and stay in your skin and fatty tissues for several months or years, and then can react with essential oils that are topically applied later. The result of the interaction can be uncomfortable side effects such as skin irritation, nausea, headaches, or the creation of chemical byproducts with unknown effects. Check Appendix B in the back of the book for other precautions when using essential oils.

I consider my skin to be fairly sensitive. I have experienced allergic reactions to such things as iodine, make-up and certain metals that jewelry is made of. I use hypoallergenic make-up and earrings. In fact, all of my personal care products are natural and as free of synthetic chemicals as I can find. As a result, in many years of personal experience with essential oils, I have never had a negative reaction. I bathe in them, wear them on my skin, use them in my hair shampoos and conditioners, and diffuse the air in my home with them.

Essential oils work well when used outside of the body and should only be taken internally under the direction and supervision of an experienced aromatherapist. Many essential oils are considered flavoring agents (FL), "Generally Regarded As Safe" (GRAS), or are certified as Food Additives (FA) by the Food and Drug Administration, and can be used as dietary supplements. A list of these oils is printed in Appendix C at the back of the book. Children under six years of age, however, should not use the oils as supplements. For anyone else taking the oils internally, they should be diluted with water, olive or vegetable oil, soy or rice milk, or mixed in food such as honey or bread. Keep in mind that the oils are very concentrated, so usually 1-2 drops taken internally during a four- to eight-hour period is effective. No more than 3 drops should be used at one time.

Are The Plant Oils Effective?

The effects of essential oils are primarily obtained through the simple act of smelling them. This may seem silly, but the fact is that the nose is one part of our "olfactory system," or the system of membranes, tissues, and nerve cells that work together with our breathing and our brain to produce the sense of smell. The nerves in the olfactory system receive electrical signals and impulses from a smell, and then, send messages to different parts of the body.

Susanne Fischer-Rizzi, a holistic healer and aromatherapy expert, pointed out in her book, *Complete Aromatherapy Handbook*, that the membranes in the nose (our "olfactory membranes") are the only part of the body that contain exposed nerves having direct contact with the environment. The olfactory membranes of our nose also contain brain cells that receive bits of information with each breath and transmit them to the nerves in our nose, and from there, to our central nervous system. So, every time we take a breath through the nose, our nervous system is activated.

Scientists have discovered that while unpleasant smells are sent to a separate part of the body, pleasant smells pass through the nasal cavity and are directed to the limbic system, or "olfactory brain." The limbic system is connected with our sexuality, likes and dislikes, motivation, moods and emotions, memory, creativity, and our autonomic nervous system (automatic functions like breathing, digestion, and heartbeat). Once in the limbic system, smells can generate the release of antibodies and neurotransmitters, like encephaline, endorphins, serotonin, and noradrenaline. According to Fischer-Rizzi, these neurotransmitters have different functions:

- Encephaline and Endorphins reduce pain and create a feeling of wellbeing;
- Encephalines also produce pleasant, euphoric sensations;
- Endorphins also stimulate sexual feelings;
- Serotonin relaxes and calms;
- Noradrenaline stimulates and makes you more alert and awake.

To list each of the several thousand chemical and aromatic elements of the oils that are identified and registered today, and their benefits, is beyond the scope of this book. However, this gives you an idea of some of their healing properties and actions on the body.

Oils For The AD/HD Diagnosis

There are many essential oils that are known for their effects on mental and emotional symptoms. Because each oil can affect many different things that are not a topic of this book, it is important to talk with an aromatherapist or to check other sources before using the oils. In the section below, I provide a sampling of oils that are viewed as calming to the body, mind, emotions and spirit. These oils can have a positive effect on many of the symptoms we describe as AD/HD:

Hyperactivity. *Valerian* and *Cedarwood* are two oils that stand out as good ones for calming the overactive child. *Lavender, Vetiver, Roman*

Chamomile, and *Peppermint* can also be tried. To use one as an inhalant, start with five times a day for up to 30 days, and then take a break for 5 days. To use them directly, apply 2-4 drops to the toes and balls of the feet as needed. Be careful when selecting a lavender oil for calming purposes. Some varieties have stimulating properties rather than calming ones. These are only examples of many possibilities. Check with an expert and your resources for other choices.

Inattention. There are certain oils that can help focus and calm the emotions and the mind. When our mind is distracted with emotional chaos, so are we. *Basil,* for example, is considered an antidepressant. It can cheer the mood and support emotional strength. *Cypress* is good for absent-mindedness and lack of concentration. *Hyssop* can help with concentration, confusion, mental clarity, and mental stimulation. *Lemongrass* can support concentration, and lift grumpiness. *Lemon Verbena* may be useful for daydreaming. Mint can ease mental fatigue, and help with concentration and clear thinking. *Peppermint* is thought to improve concentration and mental accuracy. *Rosemary* is a nerve tonic and brain stimulant that can be used to stimulate the central nervous system, strengthen memory, and support mental clarity and awareness. Some companies also make oil blends that are designed to support mental clarity and awareness. Two examples are *Brain Power* and *Clarity* made by Young Living Essential Oils.

Insomnia. Certain oils are useful when needing to create a state of inner calm for restful sleep. Examples of oils that can be used to help with difficulty sleeping are *Balm* or *Melissa, Cedarwood, Roman Chamomile, Clary Sage, Lavender, Mandarin, Neroli, Orange* or *Orange Flower Absolute,* and *Sandalwood. Roman Chamomile* is considered especially helpful for children's sleep difficulties.

Choosing Essential Plant Oils

There are many companies that produce essential oils. Essential oils are taken from plants in a number of ways. Each company has its own standards and methods for cultivating and processing the oils, so quality and purity will vary from company to company. They are also made with different degrees of purity. Purity determines the strength of an oil and affects its healing properties. Here are some things to check when choosing an oil:

1. What plant is it from? Is it from the plant that it says it is from? Check the list of ingredients on the package or bottle and contact the company if you have questions.

2. What country is it from, and does the country have the kind of growing conditions the plant needs for the best quality of oil?

3. Where were the plants grown and how? Organic plants in the wild produce the best quality oils. Avoid essential oils that come from plants grown in areas that use high amounts of chemical fertilizers and pesticides because these poisons can end up in the oil.

4. Is an expensive oil blended with less expensive ones? Or is an expensive oil made from a combination of less expensive ones? This can weaken the healing power of the oil and will not have the same effect on the body. Read the list of ingredients to see what single oils have been combined, and check individual prices to see if cheaper oils have been blended with more expensive ones. Contact the company with questions.

5. Is the oil diluted with a base of some other kind of oil like almond, grape seed, vegetable or mineral oil? These often have very little of the essential plant oil in them. Sometimes this is not listed on the label. Check your sources or the company that makes the oils you choose.

6. Does the oil have any additives in it like synthetic scents, citral, retonal or synthetic camphor? These weaken the healing power of the oil and some may even cause illness.

7. Do all the oils cost the same? This is a sign that the oils are not pure. The process for getting pure essential oil can change from plant to plant. Some are easier and some are harder, and the price reflects the differences in this process.

8.   What is the purity of the oil? Be aware that the more "pure" the oil, the more powerful is its healing ability.

Using The Oils

Direct Application. To be mindful of sensitivities, always do a skin test with an essential oil before applying it for the first time. Rub a drop or two on a small area of skin and monitor it for any reactions for an hour. Use one oil at a time when trying new products. Keep a bottle of pure vegetable oil or massage oil handy; they will dilute the oils in case of any skin irritation. Do not apply oils near the eye area or in the ears. These are sensitive areas and can become irritated from certain oils.

Here are several ways to use the oils directly:

Massage Oil: Blend 10 to12 drops of essential oil with 20 ml of massage oil (like jojoba or vegetable oil), 60 drops to 100 ml of massage oil, or 3 to 4 drops to ½ teaspoon of massage oil. Massage the oil on the body or certain parts of the body. The oils' ability to penetrate cells enables them to spread throughout the body within minutes of contact with the skin.

Warm Packs: Cover the area of the body where the essential oil was applied with a warm, dampened cloth to deepen its penetration into the skin. Cover the dampened cloth with a dry towel or blanket to hold in the heat for 15 to 30 minutes.

Bath: Mix 2 to 10 drops of essential oil with ¼ cup of your favorite (natural, non-synthetic) bubble bath, bath gel, bath salts, or Epsom salts before adding them to running bath water. Mixing the oils in this way will prevent stronger oils from irritating sensitive body areas, and will disperse the oil more evenly in the water (since oil does not mix with water).

Perfume: Dab an essential oil or oil blend on the skin as a perfume. You can put them on your wrists, feet, ear lobes, nape of the neck, nose, forehead, naval center, or anywhere else on the body. Essential oils are particularly safe and effective when used on the bottom of the feet. Some aromatherapists recommend that the oils be placed on specific points of the body that correspond with the particular aspects of the oil being used. For example, *Lavender* is a soothing oil that can be used anywhere on the body, while *Roman Chamomile* (which can also calm you down and relieve restlessness and tension) is best used on the wrists, ankles, and bottom of the feet. Check Appendix B for precautions on using stronger oils on the ears or other sensitive body areas.

Mister: Mix 2 ounces of water with 4 drops of oil and pour this into a small mister bottle. Spray your head or face as often as you want. For people with sensitive skin, this dilutes the oil and is a more gentle application than using the concentrated oil directly.

Toilet Water: Add 3 drops of essential oil to 100 ml. of distilled water to make toilet water. Use it in a bath, or splash it on after bathing as a skin freshener. Keep the mixture in a dark airtight bottle and it will stay fresh for a few weeks.

Indirect Application. If you'd rather not use them directly, oils are very effective when inhaled. There are several ways to accomplish this:

Inhalant: Carry a bottle of oil with you and sniff it as much as you want. You can also put 4 drops of oil on a small cotton cloth and carry it with you. Recharge this with 1-2 drops of oil as needed. Or, place 4 to 6 drops in the palms of your hands, rub your hands together, and then cup them over your nose and mouth while breathing deeply.

Diffuser: You can diffuse oils into the air of your home from 15 minutes and up to 2 hours a day. Keep the diffuser up high so that the oil can be misted into the air, hang around for a bit, and make its way down, taking all the unwanted particles with it. One bottle of oil can last anywhere from 8 to 48 hours, depending on its consistency. Thicker oils diffuse more slowly than thinner oils. Mixing oils is not recommended, as this can change the oil's benefits. Wash the diffuser with alcohol, natural soap and warm water before adding a new oil into it.

Cold-air diffusers are best, because heat can decrease the therapeutic quality of the oil. Cold-air diffused oils can improve air quality by reducing bacteria, fungus, mold, and unpleasant odors; aid in relaxation, relieve tension, and clear the mind; stimulate neurotransmitters and the release of endorphins in the brain; relieve headaches; improve hormone balance; help with digestion and weight management; and improve concentration, alertness, and mental clarity.

If you don't have a cold-air diffuser, you can use a spray bottle by mixing the oil with 1 cup of distilled water. Shake the bottle well before spraying the air in the room.

Vaporizer or humidifier: Place 6-8 drops of oil on a heat source, like a radiator or small bowl of hot water. To use directly on the dispenser of a vaporizer or humidifier, first add honey, sea salt, or bath salt to the water to emulsify the oils. This will help them dispense more easily. Then add 1 to 2 drops of essential oil to the water.

Essential oils can be a nice complement to other strategies you may choose to use with your child to shift behavior. The oils are safe, easy to use, and are a natural way to support the body's balance, health and functioning. Similar to essential oils, flower essences are also an easy way to safely support balance within your child's body so they can be their best every day. Read on to learn more about flower essences…

Flower Essence Remedies

What Are Flower Essences?

Dr. Edward Bach, an English physician and homeopath, is considered the modern pioneer of flower essences. However, many essences were used centuries ago in India, China, and Europe for health and healing. To create his 38 essences, Bach selected 37 wild flowers and tree blossoms with healing properties, plus one essence (Rock Water) that is derived from natural spring water. The 39th formulation (Rescue Remedy) is a combination of five essences specifically for emergencies. From the flowers, Bach developed flower essences, or tinctures (flower extracts dissolved in an alcohol and water base), that balance people's emotional states.

Modern companies have begun to expand on Bach's flower essence research. One such company is Flower Essence Services (FES). Their essences are well researched and there is documentation on using the remedies with children. There is also a company out of Australia that makes flower essences that are viewed by many professionals to be very effective. Australian Bush Flower Essences has a strong reputation for producing effective, quality essences. There are several other companies that market essences today as well. You can research them online or in a bookstore to find current sources.

How Do They Work?

Bach was a religious man who believed that wellness was based on a "complete and full union between soul, mind, and body." He believed that there were seven moods that kept people from being their true selves, including fear, uncertainty, insufficient interest in present circumstances, loneliness, oversensitivity to influences and ideas, despondency or despair, and over-care for the welfare of others. His flower essences were selected to address these seven main moods or emotions, and their subtypes, to bring them back into balance within the person. The general theory suggests that flower essences vibrate at a certain frequency and work on an energetic level to help people move past their psycho-emotional blocks, speed internal healing, and return to a state of wholeness.

Are They Safe?

The Bach company claims that anyone from newborn to the aged, as well as animals and plants, can safely use flower essences. They have no side effects, and no effect at all when taken incorrectly, so choosing and taking them yourself is safe. They are non-addictive, although they do contain alcohol. They will not interfere with the effects of pharmaceutical medications or natural agents, such as homeopathic remedies, herbal preparations, or aromatherapy oils.

Be aware that as the essences are used on a regular basis and suppressed emotions begin to surface, your child may develop temporary physical symptoms such as rashes (while toxins are cleared from the body), exhaustion, fatigue, or the awareness of repressed emotions (feelings they were previously unaware they were holding). These will disappear as balance is restored to their mental-emotional state. It's the idea that as clean water is poured into a vessel, all the old dirt and oil that has settled on the bottom begins to rise to the surface until it is washed completely out by the clean, clear water. Once this "washing out" is complete, your child's mental-emotional body will regain a state of balance and their behavior will reflect this shift.

Are They Effective?

Flower essences are meant as an addition to (rather than a replacement of) other wellness activities, such as therapy, nutritional changes, relaxation, exercise, and any other activity for improving general health. They can be used as a preventative, or to treat emotional distress and, more indirectly, the resulting symptoms. Bach believed that a person's state of health was rooted in a harmonious relationship between their mind, or moral selves, and their soul, or spiritual selves. He believed that once harmony was reestablished between the mind and the soul, the body would return to a state of health.

Flower essences are considered energy medicine, and their physical healing action is considered to be indirect. This means that rather than working directly on the physical symptoms of the body (such as aspirin for a headache), the essences work by balancing the mental and spiritual aspects of a person, so that emotional stability results. The Bach flower essences are specifically designed to clear distress within the mental, spiritual, and emotional systems of the body, which interferes with natural healing. Essentially, they promote self-healing by creating harmony among the mental, spiritual, and emotional systems of a person, which generates a healthy flow of energy throughout the body. The body begins to feel more physically healthy as these systems become more balanced and positive. Physical symptoms are slowly, gently and subtly healed in this way.

There is little "hard science" research on the effectiveness of flower essences, as specific studies have generally not been done, other than to explore the properties of the essences themselves. There is, however, testimonial data from folks who have used the essences successfully for their own healing. I am one of those folks. I keep a stash of flower remedies in my cabinet and use them for emotional issues that tend to surface now and again in my life. I have never had a negative response to an essence. What I have noticed is that when I use one on a regular basis, I will awaken one day to realize that the issue for which I was taking it has shifted. The effects are subtle and completely non-invasive. They seem to work in a very gentle yet definite way.

Flower Essences For The AD/HD Diagnosis

As with other natural agents, there are certain flower essences that can help to calm symptoms that we link to AD/HD. Some examples of these essences are presented below:

Hyperactivity. There are certain behaviors that are associated with children whose symptoms are highly externalized. These children may be viewed as high strung, argumentative, overly-enthusiastic, overly-excited, or demanding. Two Bach Flower Essences that address these behaviors are *Chicory* and *Vervain*. Chicory can help children let go of the need to be the center of attention. *Vervain* can calm hyperactivity and night-time restlessness.

Inattention. Five Bach Flower Essences stood out to me as being useful for such symptoms as inattention, difficulty listening, daydreaming, distractibility, indecision, and procrastination. These essences are *Clematis* (for the dreamy "space cadet"), *Heather* (for the self-involved), *Hornbeam* (for the mentally fatigued and overly tired),

Scleranthus (for indecision), and *White Chestnut* (for the distracted "worrywart").

Insomnia. There are two Bach Flower Essences that can help calm restlessness at night, generally due to underlying worry and anxiety. These are *Agrimony* and *White Chestnut*.

Other Essences. Australian Bush Flower Essences markets a combination remedy called "Superlearning" that is said to be of help with symptoms of AD/HD. This company and essence is worth checking into. For more information on flower remedies, refer to a full guide, such as *Bach Flower Essences for the Family*, or for more extensive information, Donna Cunningham's, *Flower Remedies Handbook*. Cunningham is a recognized author of numerous books, counselor, and expert on emotional healing with flower remedies. She began using flower remedies with her clients in 1981. You can also search the internet for companies that make flower essences and will also find information about their reputations.

Using Flower Essences

To use the flower essences or remedies, place four drops in some water or juice and drink it four times a day. Better yet, place two to four drops directly on or under the tongue for 30 seconds until absorbed, four times a day. When taken straight from the bottle, however, you will be more aware of their alcohol content. The dosage is the same for children and adults.

The action of flower essences on the body and being are gentle and subtle, as opposed to harsh and dramatic. The amount of time it takes to feel the effects of a remedy varies from person to person, and depends on the circumstances. In general, you may notice a change more quickly when dealing with situational symptoms, than when dealing with symptoms that are deeply rooted in a person. How long to use a remedy also depends on the circumstances. A person can stop using a remedy when they experience a sense of physical and emotional relief.

If a remedy is taken for 14 days without noticeable change, consider the possibility that you did not select the best match for the symptoms, and try a different remedy. If change has been minimal, it is possible that you missed some aspect of the situation, so consider adding another essence to what is already being taken. Oftentimes, new symptoms begin to surface as others are healed and cleared from the body. Healing repressed (hidden, unconscious, deeply rooted) emotions is generally a slow, steady *process*, not a one-time fix.

When Not To Use Flower Essences

Donna Cunningham believes that there are some people who should not use the remedies. For such people, the remedies are not likely to be helpful without expert guidance. These include people:

1. whose health is in a fragile or sensitive condition,
2. whose emotional state is extremely fragile,
3. who show their emotions indirectly by imagining physical illness,
4. who are heavily addicted or on powerful tranquilizers,
5. who are not ready to change, and
6. who gain something from keeping their problems.

She also discourages use by people who do not ask for the remedy themselves. This may be due to the fact that young children generally cannot identify exactly what their emotional dilemma is, or what mental-emotional symptom they are experiencing. For infants and young children, then, adults must be detectives in determining which remedy is called for.

Flower essences can be a nice addition to whatever other changes you make with your child to address their symptoms. They are a natural and subtle way to encourage deep healing of their mental-emotional being. You may also notice positive shifts in their behavior. In turn, this deep healing will support their overall functioning and long-term sense of wellness.

Are Oils And Essences Worth Trying?

In closing this chapter, let me say that everyone has an opinion about what they believe is best for children, and I can guarantee you that anyone you speak to will have an opinion about the usefulness of aromatherapy oils and flower essences. Many modern-day doctors and others working with children may judge you for even considering them as a possible option in dealing with your child's behavior. Folks who do not have any experience with oils and essences, and who have not educated themselves about them, may have their personal opinions, but that's all they are: their personal opinions.

There are experts in the fields of psychology, health and medicine who have studied the properties of these oils and essences for decades, and who do indeed know much about them. They are the folks to listen to when considering whether or not to try them with your child. What I've included in this chapter are the findings from some of these experts. My goal is to give you enough information to decide if it's something you want to look into further. You are the only one who knows what feels right to try with your child and what does not. Trust yourself, educate yourself, and then make the wisest decision you can with the information you have. That is the best you can do for your child and their long-term wellbeing.

12

WHAT PARENTS CAN DO IN A NUTSHELL

Ten guidelines to holistic parenting

As you have seen from reading this book, there are many, many ways to support your child's development. Every approach will have benefits and drawbacks, and every approach can help *someone*. How helpful an approach may be for *your* child depends on their history and profile. The key is to spend some time reviewing each area of your child's life and evaluating how healthy it is. Think about, for example, major health events, illnesses, injuries, traumas, life changes, stress, nutrition and allergies. Consider their lifestyle, routines, and typical behavior patterns. Review your parenting and relationship with them. Chances are that you will be asked about these issues when you take your child to the doctor anyway (whether allopathic or naturopathic).

The holistic approach that I favor involves supporting children in being their best on all levels. This means supporting their physical, mental, emotional, spiritual, and energetic health and development. In this way, you address the whole child, rather than just one part of the child. It also means that you must be prepared to take responsibility for not only your child's well being, but your *own*. You cannot support your child in being a whole and healthy person until you are able to do that for yourself. Be willing to take an honest look at yourself and your lifestyle, and begin to change the parts that do not add to your vitality and health. By creating a healthy life for yourself, you will be in a better position to create a healthy life for your child.

If you are reading this book, most likely you are struggling with questions about the best way to help your child be the best person they can be, now and in the future. This is one of the moments in your child's life when your time and energy are priceless to them. The effort you show in finding the most positive solution to their situation will mean everything to their long-term functioning and wellbeing. Children depend on the adults in their lives for guidance and direction. Parents and caregivers are their most important role models and their greatest allies. This is the time to make well-informed decisions about your child's health and wellbeing.

In this final chapter of the book, I offer ten guidelines to help you shift into a more holistic model of parenting. Keep in mind that this is my personal opinion. It contains biases toward a holistic, preventive and natural approach because I believe this approach holds long-term value for children. I view these guidelines as a way that adults can teach children how to make healthy lifestyle choices that foster responsibility and prevention. Rather than living haphazardly and dealing with consequences in children's physical, mental, emotional, spiritual, and energetic bodies, let's focus our attention on teaching them how to live in a healthy way. This includes not only how they manage their own bodies, but also the kind of energy they "put out" to other people and to the world around them, as these things also affect wellbeing.

Of course, it is the adults in children's lives who are their primary role models for healthful living, healthful relating, and healthful being as a member of humanity on this Earth. Basically, I believe that it is time to take responsibility for the choices we make because every choice affects ourselves, *and* the people and things around us. Let's focus our energy on creating a positive and loving space for our children to live in, and teaching them to do the same for themselves and others.

Here are ten guidelines to support you on your journey into a holistic model of wellness for your child:

1. Consider a range of treatments that starts with safer, less intrusive options and gradually moves to riskier, more intrusive alternatives as a last resort. There are many ways to address the symptoms your child may be showing. Be willing to put time and energy into exploring the different treatment choices to create a healthy, long-term solution for your child. The general model of treatment supported by child advocate organizations like The National Association of School Psychologists is to begin with the least intrusive options, and gradually move toward more intrusive options as needed. In this way, children only get exposed to harsh or severe interventions as a *last* resort. (See Chapter 2.)

By "least intrusive" I mean those interventions that carry few risks and involve the least change for the child. For example, I consider changing the way you respond to your child a mild, or least intrusive, strategy. In contrast, interventions that are "more intrusive" carry more risk and involve high amounts of change for the child. For example, having children take prescription drugs for their symptoms means putting potent chemicals into their bodies *every* day. I consider this a fairly intrusive treatment approach, especially since research suggests that they carry many health risks, even to the point of being fatal for some children.

Many parents' dilemma is that because prescription drugs contain powerful chemicals, they have an almost immediate impact on the brain and body. Since this results in rapid mood and behavioral changes in children, many people view this as a positive effect. The reality is that although these drugs may calm your child's symptoms, they are a temporary "patch." Your child's behavior will only be different while the drugs are active in their brain and body. As soon as they stop taking the drugs, their challenging behaviors return. This is because the behaviors are only a symptom, and the drugs do not cure the underlying cause of the symptoms. In fact, they mask the behavioral clues that point to a true cause.

I believe that holistic approaches are more effective than prescription medications in the long run, although they may be slower to shift things overall. I believe that they are a safer and more effective way to treat the whole child and support the health of their body, mind, emotions, and spirit/energy. Be willing to consider approaches that you believe will have the safest and most positive impact on your child's *long-term* health and functioning. Remember that the intended use for medication is within these limits:

1. if you cannot find a less-intrusive strategy that works for your child;
2. if your child's symptoms are so severe that immediate, short-term relief is needed;
3. and *always* along with other interventions (medications are intended to be used *in addition to* other treatments and never alone).

2. Create an emotionally safe environment for your child. This means allowing your child to express their feelings, as well as being mindful of how you respond to them - what you say, and how you say it. Remember that children respond to unspoken messages more than spoken ones. Your words, tone and mannerisms carry energy that send an emotional message to children (See Chapter 3). Be willing to become the most loving communicator you can with your child.

3. Review your parenting and consult a professional therapist if needed. The way you parent your child has a large impact on how they feel and behave. Shifting the way you parent is one way to change environmental factors to support your child's behavior (See Chapters 3 and 4). Be willing to take responsibility for whatever part of your parenting you may be able to adjust to ease the situation. In this way, you and your child become partners in creating a more comfortable life together, rather than the outcome resting entirely on your child's ability to change their behavior.

4. Review your family's lifestyle. Remember that doctors can treat symptoms, but you are primarily responsible for your own health, and that of your child. Optimum health requires proper nutrition, sleep, relaxation, exercise, and hygiene (See Chapters 6 and 7). Consult a naturopath or a clinical nutritionist to help with making any needed changes in these areas. Be willing to make preventive adjustments in your family's lifestyle. This is a good opportunity to teach your child about the long-term health benefits of preventive self-care practices.

5. Attend to your child's spiritual development. I do not mean "religion" here. Spiritual teachings from around the world emphasize the importance of making time to be quiet and still. This allows us to move beyond the stress of life and connect to the loving, creative energy or life force that exists in and around us. Having a connection to our Divine Source allows us to stay in loving connection to ourselves, which then enables us to have a loving connection to others and to the natural world that sustains us. This sense of connection is an important foundation from which we base our decisions and actions. When children can relate to the people and things around them with a sense of likeness or connection, they can behave in more loving and compassionate ways towards them. This will enable them to share their energy in more loving ways in the world. Be willing to have an open mind to the creative energy that science has now proven exists in and around everyone and everything. Once you open your mind to this energetic awareness, your behavior will shift, and so will your child's.

6. Review your child's exposure to mental and emotional stimulation through techno-toys. Many of today's technological toys for children are filled with messages of inappropriate sexuality, hate, anger, war, violence, aggression, cruelty, and bloodshed. Shows on television, computer games, video games, and movies, for example, have become increasingly more realistic, vulgar, sexual, and violent (See Chapter 8). Likewise, it seems that what used to be rated "R" a decade ago is rated "PG-13" today.

It does not take a scientific study to tell us that the images, sounds, and energy coming from these sources have a negative, rather than a positive, influence on the mental, emotional, behavioral, and spiritual/energetic status of children and adolescents. Remember that we recall 50% of what we see and hear (passive visual and verbal stimulation), and 90% of what we say and do (active participation). Be mindful of what you allow your children to watch and play. Be willing to take responsibility as their parent to impose healthy boundaries on their entertainment choices.

7. Consider engaging your child in therapy to learn new coping skills. Sometimes children need extra attention to develop certain social and coping skills for dealing with the world around them. Therapy provides a safe place for children to express themselves, practice newly learned skills, and get regular and immediate feedback about their behavioral choices (see Chapter 5). This takes some of the load off parents and gives children a support person that they do not have to fear losing.

When therapy ends, children learn about healthy ways to say goodbye to people they care about. This, too, is a skill, since saying goodbye to loved ones is a part of life. Therapy, whether done individually, in a group or as a family, can support the development of a healthy relationship with the self and others. Be willing to accept the guidance and support of trained professionals who have your child's best interests at heart.

8. Educate yourself about the options, risks, benefits, costs, and insurance coverage for holistic interventions. Our bodies are more aligned with the rhythms and cycles of the natural world than they are with anything else. Chapters 9 through 11 discuss several options for treating children's symptoms that work with the body's natural systems and are on the more gentle and mild end of the treatment spectrum. These include balancing the body and brain with biofeedback, chiropractic care, CranioSacral therapy, Chinese acupuncture or tui' na, and working with sensory input; and the use of natural agents such as homeopathy, herbal and Chinese medicines, essential oils, and flower essences.

Despite what some people believe, many families have had tremendous long-term success with using these so-called "alternative" and holistic methods. You might find a solution for your child's symptoms that works with their body's natural ability to harmonize and does not carry the kinds of unhealthy risks that medications do. Be willing to educate yourself about holistic options available for prevention and treatment of your child's symptoms and make a well-informed decision about what will safely serve them in being their very best in life every day.

9. Become a partner with your child's teachers. Since children spend most of their time at school, it is valuable to parents to keep a positive working relationship with school personnel. Although part of this responsibility belongs to the school, the other part of it belongs to the parents. Teachers may have thirty students to keep track of, whereas you may only have one - your own child. Take an active role and initiate school contact when you have a concern. This shows that you are prepared to be responsible for your part of the issue, and are willing to work with the school to find a solution. It also gives your child the message that you take their schooling seriously, and are willing to pay attention to what is happening in that part of their world. If you wait for the school to contact you, it may mean that things have escalated to a more serious point.

Oftentimes, the typical 15-minute conference does not allow for enough of a partnership to develop between parents and teachers. Find creative ways to stay in regular communication with school personnel about your child's progress. Let teachers know that you want to be as much a part of your child's school team as you can be, and that you are willing to participate in creating a program that will work for both your child and his or her teachers.

If you become concerned about the behavior of your child's teacher, make an appointment to talk with the teacher about it (either by phone or in person). You could also schedule a meeting with the principal, school counselor, school psychologist, or teaching team leader and invite the teacher to join you. This way, there can be no "side-stepping," "taking sides," or confusing of information, and everyone shares in the concern together as a team. Prepare yourself to speak honestly, yet calmly, and to openly listen to other points of view. Remember that you all share the same goal: for your child to make as much progress as possible in school. Be willing to consider the teachers' unique experiences with your child that may make a positive difference in planning for their success. Keep in mind that your child's behavior may be very different in school than it is at home. Be willing to listen openly to the school's unique point of view.

10. Consider a broadened view of children's health. When thinking about what is best for your child's long-term growth and development, it may be necessary to broaden the way you think about general health. I believe that human health is the product of a combination of personal, social, and environmental factors. This means that your child's health is affected not only by their physical makeup, but by how well they take care of themselves, and by how they interact with the world around them. Although you have no control over your child's genetic makeup, you *do have* control over their self-care and how they interact with the outside environment.

What I am proposing here is that to approach health and life holistically, your attention is given to a triad of focus that includes the self, others and the environment. By teaching children to take responsibility for how they live their lives in terms of self-care, other-care, and what I call Earth-care, you can impact their health and wellbeing in life-long, positive ways. Although I discussed some of these ideas earlier in the book, I feel they are worth repeating here:

Self-Care. Since children are not in a position to take complete care of themselves, health is largely determined by the lifestyle of their parents and caregivers. That is why it is so important for parents and caregivers to model healthy living and self-care for children. There are many self-care things that you can do for your children and your family to prevent health issues from emerging. You read about some of these in Chapters 6, 7 and 8. Basically, this means making sure you and your family:

1. practice good hygiene;
2. eat nutritious foods;
3. drink 48 ounces of water a day;
4. sleep soundly for six to eight hours a night;
5. exercise for 20 minutes, at least three days a week;
6. limit exposure to techno-violence, aggression, and sexualized behavior;
7. make time to relax, unwind, and rebuild;
8. find ways to nurture the inner creative self and spirit; and
9. get annual health check-ups.

Healthy living also means *not* doing certain things, such as:

1. under- or over-eating;
2. under- or over-sleeping

3. under- or over-exercising
4. spending more than two hours a day watching T.V., videos, etc.
5. eating or drinking high amounts of processed foods and beverages containing large doses of sugar and fat;
6. smoking cigarettes;
7. drinking high amounts of alcohol;
8. using illegal substances;
9. ingesting high amounts of caffeine; and
10. getting too much sun exposure.

These are important health factors that you *can* control for yourself and your child, and things that you can teach them to manage in healthy ways in their own life.

Relating to others. The second part of the health triad is how your child relates to other people. As their parent and caregiver, the way you relate to others and the world around *you* largely determines how your child relates to others and the world around *them*. The quality of their social relationships is one of the foundations of staying healthy. Relationships that are loving, supportive, encouraging, safe, understanding, and accepting of who they are enhance their state of wellbeing. The positive energy that comes from them adds vitality to their body and spirit.

On the other hand, relationships that are hateful, hurtful, judgmental, critical, punitive, and rejecting weaken their state of wellbeing. The negative energy that comes from these types of relationships takes vitality away from their body and spirit. This is especially true for children who have fewer coping skills to deal with negative energy than adults do. As with lifestyle issues, it is important that parents and caregivers model positive relationships for children, so children learn to both seek out and create healthy relationships in their own lives as they grow up.

Relating to the Earth. Finally, the third part of the health triad involves the quality of your child's relationship to the Planet Earth. The topic of Earth-care is a book unto itself, so I will not spend much time on it here. What I want to emphasize is that each of us -- including your child -- has control over how we tend to the Earth and her "bounty."

Without the Earth's bounty, none of us will have health or can sustain life on this planet. When the Earth's bounty becomes polluted, everything that sustains us becomes polluted, too. There is not always "more where that came from."

To explain further, consider that the Earth is a living system. She is created in a perfect state of harmony, just as our bodies are. She provides us with everything we need to thrive. We are all "symbionts" with the Earth, meaning that we live in a relationship with her that is beneficial to each of us. We take care of her, and she takes care of us. When we stop taking care of her, she will not be able to take care of us. If we continue to pollute the Earth's soils, air, water, food and balance, there will be nothing left in a healthy state for us to survive on. We are already dealing with detoxifying certain areas of the Earth's resources. In other words, as long as the Earth is healthy and her bounty is healthy, our bodies can be healthy. The more polluted and out of balance the Earth's systems become, the more polluted and out of balance her bounty becomes, and the more polluted and out of balance our bodies become.

For this reason, I believe that it is all of our responsibility to be stewards (or caretakers) of the bounty that the Earth offers us for healthy living. Your child can learn to value and care for the Earth just as easily as they can learn to value and care for anything else in their lives. I believe that Earth care is just as critical to children's health as what they eat, drink, and do. I believe this because what they eat, drink and do will not matter if the Earth's bounty is nutritionally empty or toxic for them. Again, this is something you *can* control to ensure good health not only for yourself and your children, but also for their children and for all the future generations that will live here after us.

Here are some ways to teach children about good stewardship of the Earth:

1. **Teach them not to litter.** It is a form of pollution and carries a hefty fine in most states. Dispose of your trash in a trashcan instead of leaving it as litter on the ground. Be responsible about this around your own home, and in your community as well. An easy way to do this is to carry a small plastic bag with you when you take walks so you can pick up and recycle trash you find along the way (like metal cans or glass and plastic bottles).

Things like metal cans and glass left on the ground are not only unsightly, they can cut or otherwise hurt a person or an animal. They also tend not to biodegrade. Luckily, they can be easily recycled in most areas.

2. **Teach your children to recycle.** Today, you can recycle paper, newspapers, magazines, books, glass, plastic, cans/metal, and cardboard. You can cash in aluminum cans, and in some states, glass bottles. Many communities now have curbside recycling to make it as easy and convenient as possible, but they may not take everything. Do a little research to find the nearest recycling plant to your home and what they take. Not only does this cut down on the amount of trash you have, but it also saves resources and decreases landfill pollution.

3. **Teach your children to be mindful of their own chemical usage and the value of a lifestyle that aims to be toxic-free.** Even something as simple as perfume contains chemicals that are toxic. For instance, a chemical known as "toluene" is found in most body fragrances available in stores. This chemical is considered very toxic and can lead to headaches, nausea, and narcosis. For more information about health issues linked to chemicals, visit www.ourlittleplace.com/mcs.html, a Web site with information about "Multiple Chemical Sensitivity," which is a subset of symptoms from "Environmental Illness" resulting from living in a chemically toxic world. A list of a few of the more common fragrance toxins and what symptoms they can cause is provided here for your quick reference:

Chemical Name	Associated Symptoms
Toluene	Can cause headaches, nausea, and narcosis (stupor, unconsciousness, or arrested activity)
Musk Ambrette	Can cause central & peripheral nervous system damage

Linalool	Can provoke "ataxic" gait (lack of muscular coordination when walking), reduced motor activity, depression, respiratory problems
Methylethylketone	Can cause stupor, emphysema, congestion of the liver and kidneys
Propylene Glycol	Toxic to the immune system

4. **Use natural health care and cleaning products in your home.** Avoid products that contain such chemicals as DEA, Propylene Glycol, Sodium Lauryl Sulfate (SLS), Sodium Laureth Sulfate (SLES), talc, alcohol, and aluminum. These are found in common products such as body powder, mouthwash, bubble bath, cream, shampoo, conditioner, and toothpaste. They have been linked to things like cancer and other health issues and diseases.

   Instead, consider the many Earth-friendly personal care and household products on the market today that work as well or better than traditional, toxic ones. For instance, natural toothpaste, shampoo, soap, makeup, and cream are available in almost every grocery store. White vinegar, baking soda, and hydrogen peroxide are good for cleaning everything from mold, mildew and blood to glass surfaces and clothes. If you cannot find natural, Earth-friendly products in the general grocery stores near you, find a health food store or visit www.gaiam.com to check out some products they sell. The little bit of extra expense goes a long way in terms of self- and Earth-care.

5. **Support companies and products that believe in clean living.** Visit www.greenpages.org to access Co-Op America's *National Green Pages*, which is an Earth-friendly version of the yellow pages. You will find all kinds of "green" or environ-

mentally-safe goods and services by Earth-friendly companies.

6. **Support organic, toxic-free ranching and farming methods.** Research continues to show that man-made fertilizers, pest-control products, and quantity-increasing substances used on large-scale ranches and farms distort and degrade the quality of our food and environment. Choosing to buy organic, toxin-free foods when possible supports a healthier, sustainable food supply and environment, which is necessary for humans, animals, and plants. Although slightly more expensive, these products pay off in the long run by promoting our long life and health.

7. **Use nontoxic pesticides in your home and yard.** This is not only cleaner for the environment, but safer for you, your family, your pets, and your wildlife. For more information, visit the Texas Pesticide Information Network (or "Texas PIN") at www.texascenter.org/txpin. This Web site was developed in 1998 to provide a better public understanding of how pesticides are used in Texas and how they affect human health and the environment. It also has links to other sources of information related to pesticides and health.

8. **Save water and money by using your water smartly.** Clean water is a necessary resource for our survival. There are some very simple ways to practice water preservation and conservation. Here are a few ideas:

   - take short showers instead of long ones or baths;
   - use water efficient, low-flow showerheads;
   - install efficient, low-flow aerators on bathroom and kitchen sinks;
   - install water efficient or air assisted toilets;
   - match the water level on your washer to the size of your laundry load;
   - turn off faucets while shaving, brushing teeth, and washing hands;

- soak produce and dishes for rinsing rather than running water over them;
- thaw frozen foods in a container of hot water rather than running water over them;
- fill the dishwasher before running it;
- insulate your hot water pipes to cut down on "wait time" for hot water;
- keep your water heater temperature as low as possible; and
- repair drips and leaks immediately.

For more information and ideas, visit www.watersmart.org Web site or the Texas Water Development Board (TWDB) Web site at www.twdb.state.tx.us. The TWDB site has a "TWDB Kids" link that opens a kid-friendly page with information and educational activities for youngsters. It also has several links for adults who want more information about where their water comes from and what influences its quantity and quality.

It is important to remember that *we do not live in a vacuum*. Each of us is one player in a whole group called the Human Race, living on one part of a larger system we call the Earth, that is one planet in a vast solar system we call the Universe. We can no longer pretend that what we do in our part of the world in our lifetime does not affect those around us or those coming after us. It *does*. There is no denying that; current science supports this reality.

It is time for us to stop thinking in terms of "I" and begin thinking in terms of "We." Part of shifting into an Earth-care mentality is the ability to shift from thinking about the individual to thinking about the larger (world) group that we are each a part of. The natural cycles of the Earth are set up to work in a certain kind of harmony that we may never completely understand. Our lack of understanding, however, does *not* give us permission to disrespect or disregard the delicacy of this harmony. Our health depends on it. Our lives depend on it. Our future depends on it. Children can be taught the importance of these principles, and can join adults in making them a natural part of their lifestyle.

AD/HD Generation: Closing Comments

Children with a diagnosis of AD/HD are *everywhere*. You can rarely escape a conversation with parents without the topic of AD/HD surfacing. Although I do not believe that AD/HD is a true disorder, I know that the symptoms exist; clearly, they *do*. Many people's lives are impacted by the symptoms every day. I am not saying that there are no symptoms. What I *am* saying is that the symptoms we so readily label as AD/HD can be linked to many different factors, and in my opinion, cannot be justifiably lumped into one "AD/HD" category. Symptoms such as these are too dependent on each individual child's profile to treat them all the same.

My hope is that at this point in the book, you are willing to consider the possibility that the symptoms we call AD/HD can best be sorted out and managed on an *individual* basis founded on a holistic health model. This is in sharp contrast to viewing them as a disease or disorder to be managed on a group basis founded on the medical or allopathic "diagnose and medicate" model.

What I have presented to you in this book is complex in some ways, and simply common sense in other ways. I believe that we are in a phase of living that requires us to reevaluate and revisit the way we view health. What we need, in my opinion, is a society that supports prevention and healthy living, and a system of health care that allows each person to choose for themselves the type of care they prefer. These statements are nothing new; they are not new ideas. When you begin to really study health in our society, however, you become aware of the fact that it is an issue that reaches well beyond the individual level and into the societal, political and even global levels because it is largely about the business of money. This subject alone could be an entire book.

This is how I hope you will think about the issue of health and AD/HD from now on: not just personally, but on a larger and broader level. After all, none of us lives in a vacuum. It is not just a few children being treated with medication. It is an entire *generation* of children – an AD/HD generation of children – millions of them taking drugs daily for their behavior. This book is intended to provide you with information to begin to shift not only the way you view AD/HD, but also the way you view health and prevention in general. The children of today are counting on you – their parents – to speak out for them. They are counting on you to be their best advocate and their strongest supporter. They are counting on you to find the healthiest solutions to their challenges, and expose them to the least amount of risk. They are counting on you to love them enough to be a responsible, healthy parent invested in their future. After all, they are worth it.

APPENDIX A
OVERLAPPING SYMPTOMS OF AD/HD WITH OTHER ISSUES

Symptoms	Alternative Diagnosis				
	ADHD (DSM-IV)	Sensory Integration Dysfunction (Ayres)	Learning-related Visual Problems (Kavner)	Nutrition Allergies (Rapp, Crook, & Smith)	Normal Child Under 7 (Gesell)
Inattention					
Often fails to give close attention to details or makes careless mistakes	✓	✓	✓	✓	
Often has difficulty sustaining attention in tasks or play	✓	✓	✓	✓	✓
Often does not listen when spoken to directly	✓	✓	✓	✓	
Often does not follow through on instructions or fails to finish work	✓	✓	✓	✓	✓
Often has difficulty organizing tasks and activities	✓	✓	✓	✓	✓

Symptoms	Alternative Diagnosis				
	ADHD (DSM-IV)	Sensory Integration Dysfunction (Ayres)	Learning-related Visual Problems (Kavner)	Nutrition Allergies (Rapp, Crook, & Smith)	Normal Child Under 7 (Gesell)
Often avoids, dislikes or is reluctant to engage in tasks requiring sustained mental effort	✓	✓	✓	✓	✓
Often loses things	✓	✓	✓	✓	✓
Often distracted by extraneous stimuli	✓	✓	✓	✓	✓
Often forgetful in daily activities	✓	✓	✓	✓	
Hyperactivity & Impulsivity					
Often fidgets with hands or feet or squirms in seat	✓	✓	✓	✓	✓
Often has difficulty remaining seated when required to	✓	✓	✓	✓	✓

Symptoms	Alternative Diagnosis				
	ADHD (DSM-IV)	Sensory Integration Dysfunction (Ayres)	Learning-related Visual Problems (Kavner)	Nutrition Allergies (Rapp, Crook, & Smith)	Normal Child Under 7 (Gesell)
Often runs or climbs excessively	✓	✓		✓	✓
Often has difficulty playing quietly	✓	✓		✓	
Often "on the go"	✓	✓		✓	✓
Often talks excessively	✓	✓	✓	✓	
Often blurts out answers to questions before they have been completed	✓	✓	✓	✓	
Often has difficulty awaiting their turn	✓	✓	✓	✓	✓
Often interrupts or intrudes on others	✓	✓	✓	✓	✓

* Note: Adapted from Patricia S. Lemer, M.Ed. (2002). Attention Deficits: A Developmental Approach, p. 2-3. Available at www.devdelay.org/adhd.htm.

APPENDIX B
PRECAUTIONS FOR USING
ESSENTIAL OILS

1. Since pure, high-quality essential oils are highly concentrated and are made up of a mix of chemicals, it is best to consult a specialist who can guide you in selecting and using the right one(s) for your needs. Check with a naturopathic doctor, aromatherapy specialist, experts in the holistic store that sells the oils, or a reputable distribution company for referrals and information.

2. As with all chemical products, keep your essential oils where infants and children cannot reach them. Although natural, they are chemicals, are highly concentrated, and can have toxic and severe effects if used incorrectly. If more than five drops of an essential oil are ingested at once, contact the poison control center (1-800-764-7661) or your holistic doctor immediately.

3. Some experts recommend not using oils that are rich in menthol on the throat or neck area of children younger than 2 ½ years of age.

4. Some oils will irritate the eyes or ears, or can damage contact lenses, especially those with a high phenol content (such as oregano, helichrysum, cinnamon, thyme, clove, lemongrass, and bergamot). Be careful not to rub your eyes or ears, or handle contact lenses if you have oils on your fingers.

5. It is a good idea to skin test essential oils before using them, especially for children with sensitive skin. Remember that we are all unique and our bodies will respond differently. To skin test an essential oil, put one at a time on a part of the body with thin skin, such as under the arms, on the wrists, or behind the knees. Wait at least 15 to 30 minutes for the body to respond. If a rash develops, dilute the spot with a neutral oil such as vegetable oil.

6. Be aware of sun exposure when using essential oils. Certain ones can cause rash or darker skin coloration if exposed to direct sunlight within 3 to 4 days of use (e.g., Lemon, Bergamot, Orange, Grapefruit, Tangerine, White Angelica, and other citrus oils). This holds true for sunlamps, tanning beds, etc. as well.

7. Some oils have hormone-like effects, such as Clary Sage, Sage, Idaho Tansy, Juniper, and Fennel. Consult a specialist before using them.

8. People with a history of epilepsy or high blood pressure should consult a specialist before using oils. Avoid using Hyssop, Fennel, and Idaho Tansy.

9. Store your essential oils out of the light and/or in a dark-colored glass bottle with a tightly sealed top. They can keep their potency for years when properly stored.

Appendix C
Essential Oils That Can Be Used As Dietary Supplements

Anise	GRAS	FA	Mandarin	GRAS	FA
Angelica	GRAS	FA	Marjoram	GRAS	FA
Basil	GRAS	FA	Melaleuca Alternifolia		FA
Bergamot	GRAS	FA	Melissa (Lemonbalm	GRAS	FA
Cajeput		FA	Mountain Savory		FA
Cardamom		FA	Myrrh	(FL) GRAS	FA
Carrot Seed		FA	Myrtle	GRAS	FA
Cassia	GRAS	FA	Neroli	GRAS	FA
Cedarwood		FA	Nutmeg	GRAS	FA
Celery Seed	GRAS	FA	Onycha	GRAS	FA
Chamomile, Roman	GRAS	FA	Orange	GRAS	FA
Chamomile, German	GRAS	FA	Oregano	GRAS	FA
Cinnamon Bark/Leaf	GRAS	FA	Palmarosa	GRAS	FA
Cistus		FA	Patchouli	(FL) GRAS	FA
Citronella	GRAS	FA	Pepper	GRAS	FA
Citrus rinds (All)	GRAS	FA	Peppermint	GRAS	FA
Clary Sage	GRAS	FA	Petitgrain	GRAS	FA
Clove	GRAS	FA	Pine	(FL) GRAS	FA
Copaiba	GRAS	FA	Rosemary Cineol	GRAS	FA
Coriander	GRAS	FA	Rose	GRAS	FA
Cumin	GRAS	FA	Rosewood		FA
Dill	GRAS	FA	Savory	GRAS	FA
Eucalyptus Globulus	(FL) GRAS	FA	Sage	GRAS	FA
Elemi	(FL) GRAS	FA	Sandalwood	(FL) GRAS	FA
Fennel	GRAS	FA	Spearmint	GRAS	FA
Fir, Balsam		FA	Spikenard		FA
Frankincense	(FL) GRAS	FA	Spruce	(FL) GRAS	FA
Galbanum	(FL) GRAS	FA	Tangerine	GRAS	FA
Geranium	GRAS	FA	Tarragon	GRAS	FA
Ginger	GRAS	FA	Thyme	GRAS	FA
Grapefruit	GRAS	FA	Tsuga	(FL) GRAS	FA
Helichrysum	GRAS	FA	Valerian	(FL) GRAS	FA
Hyssop	GRAS	FA	Vetiver	GRAS	FA
Jasmine	GRAS	FA	Wintergreen		FA
Juniper	GRAS	FA	Yarrow		FA
Laurus Nobille	GRAS	FA	Ylang Ylang	GRAS	FA
Lavender	GRAS	FA			
Lavendin	GRAS	FA		Code	
Lemon	GRAS	FA			
Lemongrass	GRAS	FA	**(FL)** = Flavoring Agent		
Lime	GRAS	FA	**GRAS** = Generally Regarded As Safe		
			FA = FDA-approved food additive		

Adapted from the Essential Oils Desk Reference, pg. 485; Essential Science Publishing

APPENDIX D
WHERE TO GET MORE INFORMATION

Web Resources For Parents

Alliance: Parent Training & Information Centers and Community Parent Resource Centers
PACER CENTER
8161 Normandale Blvd.
(952) 838-9000 (voice)
(952) 838-0190 (TTY)
(852) 838-0199 (Fax)
1-888-248-0822 (Toll Free)
www.taalliance.org (web address)
alliance@taaliance.org (Email)
This group provides training and information to parents of children with disabilities, and the professionals who work with them.

Arctic Tern Publishing Company
www.arcticternpublishing.com
This web site contains medication fact sheets that provide a brief overview of different medications. They are written by Dr. Dean E. Konopasek to provide people with user-friendly, jargon-free information. Each sheet tells what the medication is used for, what it does, what side effects it has, and what the dosage range is. The sheets can be ordered for $22.95 a copy, with a 10% discount if you order multiple copies.

Children and Adults with Attention-Deficit/Hyperactivity Disorder (CHADD)
8181 Professional Place, Suite 201
Landover, Maryland 20785
(301) 306-7070
1-800-233-4050
www.chadd.org
CHADD provides support and information to families with adults or children dealing with AD/HD. Their website has "facts sheets" with

what they consider the latest information about AD/HD, including treatment options. They have little experience or information on "alternative" therapies, but do recommend a comprehensive approach along with medication.

Children's Environmental Health Network
Children's Environmental Health Coalition
110 Maryland Avenue NE, Suite 511
Washington, DC 20002
(202) 543-4033
(202) 543-8797 (FAX)
www.cehn.org

The mission of this Network and Coalition is to protect the fetus and the child from environmental health hazards, and to promote a healthy environment. Their site "provides information on the Network, the issue of children's environmental health, and links to sources of information and resources in the field." You can contact them with questions and comments at the address and phone above. You can search the site by organization name or toxicant, learn about research initiatives, and find out what resources are in your area. They also have a link to US policy on Children's Environmental Health.

Journal of Neurotherapy
www.snr-jnt.org

This site provides a list of practitioners in the U.S. (and the world). You can also read major articles on the topic of neurotherapy.

Mothers and Others for a Livable Planet
Wendy Gordon, Executive Director
40 West 20th Street
New York, NY 10011
(888) ECO-INFO
(212)242-0545 (FAX)
www.mothers.org/mothers

Mothers and Others is a national, nonprofit education organization that boasts 20,000 members. According to their website, they work to promote "consumer choices that are safe and ecologically sustainable for current and future generations." This site has links to resources with lists of organizations, data sources, educational materials, general information and fact sheets, journals, etc. They provide information on how to get involved, and a place for your comments. See www.mothers.org/tenfoods.html for a list of their top ten fruits and vegetables to buy organic according to the amount of toxicity of pesticide residues they found in them (from their newsletter, *Green Guide* #80, June, 2000).

National Attention Deficit Disorder Association (ADDA)
1788 Second Street, Suite 200
Highland Park, Illinois 60035
(847) 432-2332
www.add.org
From this website, you can link to AD/HD organizations in your area.

The National Information Center for Children & Youth with Disabilities
NICHCY
P.O. Box 1492
Washington, DC 20013
1-800-695-0285
www.nichcy.org
This center provides information on disabilities and disability-related issues to families, educators, and other professionals. They focus on ages birth to 22 years. You can call their 1-800 number and get answers to your questions. Their website has a Spanish site link with materials in Spanish. On their website, you can search through state resource sheets to help you find the organizations in your state that can help you, including agencies for youngsters, parent groups, and parent training and information.

Natural Medicines Comprehensive Database
www.naturaldatabase.com
This site has many uses. It is continuously updated, and is recognized as the standard for evidence-based information on medicine.

They cover conventional, complementary, alternative, and integrative medicine. You can get information on specific products, get a "patient handout" for a product, check research article summaries, and find out about drug interactions and safety concerns. There is a special window that gives reliable information using easy-to-understand language for patients.

The ADD/ADHD Newsletter
www.attentiondeficitdisorder.ws

This site contains five areas of information: 1) The complete AD/HD information library; 2) AD/HD product reviews and research; 3) The complete AD/HD bookstore; 4) 500 AD/HD classroom interventions; and 5) nutraceutical (natural) medicine and AD/HD. You can learn something and scan resources for more information on this site. I do not know who creates it, or if it promotes certain products.

Web Resources For Holistic Health

American Botanical Council (ABC)
1-800-373-7105
www.herbalgram.org

The ABC is a non-profit, research and educational organization created by Mark Blumenthal. It was formed in 1988 to provide non-bias information about herbs and herbal products to the public. The site contains valuable resource leads, but little on-site information about herbal medicine. If you call them, you can receive *The ABC Clinical Guide to Herbs* book.

Bach Flower Remedies, Ltd. and the Bach Center
www.bachflower.com

This site provides a description of each of the 38 remedies and their uses. There is also an on-line consultation option for quick answers to your questions.

The Biofeedback Certification Institute of America (BCIA)
10200 West 44th Avenue, Suite 304
Wheatridge, CO 80033
(303) 420-2902
www.bcia.org
This group has a directory that lists biofeedback therapists, their background and clinical experience. Call and you can get the names of practitioners in your area. Their membership organization is the Association for Applied Psychophysiology and Biofeedback. They are at the same address, but have their own membership directory, phone (303)422-8436, and website (www.aapb.org).

Herbal Materia Medica
www.healthy.net
This is a comprehensive site that has information and references on natural choices for children's health, including herbal medicine, homeopathy, osteopathy, naturopathy, integrative medicine, healthy vaccinations, and an on-line bookstore. There is a special window for AD/HD and alternative therapies.

Herbal Remedies
www.healthyideas.com/healing/herb
This site offers information about herbs and supplements for AD/HD and other health issues.

Homeopathy: Natural Health Care
http://www.homeopathy-cures.com
You can get a list of practitioners by state on this site, created by two Naturopathic Doctors in Denver, Colorado.

Medicinal Herbs Online
www.egregore.com
This site has information about medicinal herbs. They also provide a newsletter, resources, links, and an on-line bookstore and health store. They have herbal information for specific diseases, but when I checked, not AD/HD (perhaps due to the controversy over whether or not it is a disease).

National Center for Homeopathy
801 North Fairfax Street, Suite 306
Alexandria, VA 22314
(703)548-7790
www.homeopathic.org
This organization can provide you with information about homeopathy, and a list of practitioners by name, city, state, and country to help you in your searching.

Holistic Book Resources

The ADHD Parenting Handbook: Practical Advice for Parents from Parents **(1994). Colleen Alexander-Roberts. Taylor Publishing Company: Dallas, TX.**
This book offers parents useful ideas about how to deal with challenging behavior without drugs. For example, chapters 5, 6, and 7 address handling problems that "drive you wild," ways to prevent misbehavior, and working with your child's teachers and school.

ADD: It Doesn't Add Up! Drug-Free Alternatives For Hyperactivity & Aggression **(1997). Susan Stockton. Nature's Publishing & Printing: Murdock, FL.**
This is a good resource for learning about food allergies and sensitivities, as well as nutritional links to the symptoms of AD/HD. It is a very user-friendly booklet that parents will find helpful.

A.D.D. The Natural Approach **(1996). Nina Anderson & Howard Peiper. Safe Goods. East Canaan, CT.**
This is an easy-to-read booklet providing valuable information about nutrition and how it is linked to the symptoms of AD/HD. They also touch on other natural alternative therapies, including Aromatherapy, Chinese Medicine, CranioSacral Therapy, flower remedies, and herbal medicine. They provide two resource lists: one for nutritional supplements, and one for recommended books.

Earthlight: New Meditations For Children **(1997). Maureen Garth. HarperCollins Publishers: New York.**

This is an excellent resource for children's meditations and creative visualizations. Maureen also published a meditation book for teenagers called, *InnerSpace,* and one for adults called, *The Power of the Inner Self.* I recommend them all.

Essential Oils Desk Reference, Fourth Edition (2007). Essential Science Publishing. *www.essentialscience.net.*
This desk reference contains everything you need to know about essential oils and how they can be used for health and healing.

Flower Remedies Handbook: Emotional Healing & Growth with Bach & Other Flower Essences, (1992). Donna Cunningham. Sterling Publishing Co., Inc.: New York.
This book contains good information about essential oils and how to use them for emotional healing. It is easy to understand and fairly comprehensive. Cunningham includes a list of several companies that make flower essences with a description of each, including an appendix of which ones supply specific remedies. She is a counselor with a Master's Degree in social work who has used flower essences to support emotional balance with her clients for more than 15 years.

Releasing Emotional Patterns with Essential Oils (1998). Carolyn L. Mein, D.C.
This book describes ways of clearing emotional patterns from the body's cellular memory with essential oils. Our bodies hold emotions in the glands and organs. This emotional energy can be released from the body by using the oils on acupuncture points of the body and through the limbic system, which is accessed with smell.

The Myth of the ADD Child (1995). Thomas Armstrong. Dutton Publishers: New York.
This book provides readers with an interesting review of what Thomas Armstrong calls the AD/HD myth, plus 50 ways to improve your child's behavior and attention without medication. It is full of valuable information for any parent who chooses to empower their children, rather then control them.

References

ADD-Information.com (2001), ADD - Relief for Attention Deficit Disorder - Treatment without drugs. www.healing-arts.org/children/ADHD/herbal.htm.

Alan Agnins, Ph.D. *Herbal and Natural Supplements: Their Use in Children and Adolescents.* An excerpt from A Guide to Common Medical Conditions & Drugs Used in School-Aged Children. Manisses Communications Group, Inc.: Providence, RI. www.manisses.com

Nina Anderson & Howard Peiper (1996). A.D.D.: The Natural Approach. Safe Goods: East Canaan, CT.

Dr. Thomas Armstrong (1995), The Myth of the A.D.D. Child, Plume: NY.

Virginia M. Axline (1947). Play Therapy, Ballantine Books, Publishers: NY.

Bach Flower Essences (2000). Bach Flower Essences for the Family: An introduction to the basic principles and standards of the Bach Flower essences and a guide to their use. Wigmore Publications, Ltd.: London, Great Britain.

Stephen Barr (January, 1999). Computer violence: Are your kids at risk? Special report in Reader's Digest.

A. Benner (1979). Trace mineral levels in hyperactive children responding to the Feingold diet. Journal of Pediatrics, vol. 94(6).

Boiron (Date unknown). The Smart Guide to Homeopathy. Boiron. Newtown Square, PA. Telephone: 1-800-BOIRON-1 (264-7661).

M. Boris & F. Mandel (1994). Foods and additives are common causes of the Attention Deficit Hyperacticity Disorder in Children. Annals of Allergy, vol. 72.

Joan Breakey (1997). Review Article, The role of diet and behavior in childhood. Journal of Pediatric Child Health, vol. 33.

Ana Brett & Ravi Singh (2007). Kundalini Yoga for Beginners & Beyond. Raviana Productions. www.raviana.com.

Sheila Bullock (1992). Homeopathy: What is it? Superior Printing: Dallas, TX.

Bonnie W. Camp, M.D., Ph.D. (Summer, 1996). "Think Aloud," Communique', National Association of School Psychologists, Publishers.

Peter Chappell (1994). Emotional Healing with Homoeopathy. Element: Boston, Massachusetts.

John O. Cooper, Timothy E. Heron, & William L. Heward (1987). Applied Behavior Analysis, Merrill Publishing Company: Columbus, Ohio.

Dr. Tom Cushman & Dr. Thomas Johnson (2000). Nutritional, Medical and Ecological Sources of Inattention. Communique', V29 (3).

Dr. Richard DeGrandpre (2000, 1999). Ritalin Nation: Rapid-fire Culture and the Transformation of Human Consciousness. W.W. Norton & Company: NY.

Don Dinkmeyer & Gary McKay (1989). STEP (Systematic Training for Effective Parenting): The Parent's Handbook. STEP Publishers, LLC. See STEPforParents.com.

T. Druckman & A. Minevich (1998), "Applications of EEG - Neurofeedback for Attention Deficit Disorder," webideas.com/biofeedback/research.minevich.htm.

Dr. James Duke (1997). The Green Pharmacy; Rodale Press: Emmaus, PA.

John Dye, Naturopathic Doctor (ND) (2000), "Herbal Medicine and Treatments for Attention-Deficit/Hyperactivity Disorder (ADHD)," on the web at www.healing-arts.org/children/ADHD/herbal.htm.

Rita Elkins, M.H. (Sept., 2001). ADHD: Help Drug Free. Great Life Magazine.

Dr. Kevin Ross Emery (2000). Managing the gift: alternative approaches for attention deficit disorder. LightLines Publishing, NH.

Essential Oils Desk Reference, Fourth Edition (2007). Essential Science Publishing.   ·

Susanne Fischeri-Rizzi (1990), Complete Aromatherapy Handbook: Essential Oils for Radiant Health. Sterling Publishing Co., Inc.: NY.

Leo Galland, M.D. (1988). Superimmunity for Kids: What to feed your children to keep them healthy now, and prevent disease in the future. Dell Publishing, NY.

Stephen W. Garber, Ph.D., Marianne Daniels Garber, Ph.D., & Robyn Freedman Spizman (1996). Beyond Ritalin: Facts About Medication and Other Strategies for Helping Children, Adolescents, and Adults with Attention Deficit Disorders. Harper Perennial: NY.

Maureen Garth (1997). Earthlight: New Meditations For Children. HarperCollins Publishers: New York.

Howard Glasser (February 2002). Workshop entitled, "Transforming the Difficult Child", based on the book, Transforming the Difficult Child (1998), by Howard Glasser and Jennifer Easley, Center for the Difficult Child Publications: Tucson, AZ. www.difficultchild.com.

Daniel Goleman, Ph.D., & Joel Gurin (Editors) (1993). Mind Body Medicine: How to Use Your Mind for Better Health. Consumer Reports Books: Yonkers, NY.

Robert J. Goodman. "Attention Deficit Disorder (ADD) and the Atlas Subluxation Complex" in The Upper Cervical Monograph. Goodman is a Doctor of Chiropractic and a member of NUCCA.

Dr. Thomas Gordon (1975). P.E.T., Parent Effectiveness Training: The Tested New Way To Raise Responsible Children, Plume, Publishers: NY.

Lt. Col. Dave Grossman (1995). On killing: The psychological cost of learning to kill in war and society. A BACK BAY BOOK.

David Hoffman (1988). The Herbal Handbook: A User's Guide to Medical Herbalism. Healing Arts Press: Rochester, VT.

David Hoffman (1996), The Complete Illustrated Holistic Herbal. Barnes & Noble Books, NY.

Joan Horton & Jenni Zimmer (1994), "Media Violence and Children: A guide for parents," brochure developed by the National Association for the Education of Young Children.

Dr. Judy J. Hughes (2002). "Is Your Bright Child Struggling in School?" Center for Vision Improvement; www.austineyegym.com.

International Chiropractic Pediatric Association (2001). "ADD/ADHD," www.4icpa.org/research/add.htm.

Lynda Kirk (March 1996). "EEG Biofeedback and ADD;" Austin Monthly Magazine.

Patricia S. Lemer, M.Ed. (1995). Attention Deficits: A Developmental Approach. www.devdelay.org/adhd.htm.

Jennifer E. Lingenfelter (2001). Review of the literature regarding the efficacy of neurofeedback in the treatment of Attention Deficit Hyperactivity Disorder. Doctoral Research Paper, Biola University. ERIC#ED457634.

Lynn Lott, M.A., M.F.C.C., & Jane Nelsen, Ed.D., M.F.C.C. (1988). Teaching Parenting the Positive Discipline Way, p. 101. Printed in the U.S. To order, call toll-free: 1-800-456-7770; or write to Empowering People Books, Tapes & Videos, P.O. Box 1926, Orem, UT, 84059.

Maharishi Vedic Education Development Corporation (1999). "The TM program & ADHD"; http://users.erols.com/tmdelco/page5.html.

Dr. Siegfried Othmer (1998), "Mental fitness training for attention, learning, and behavior problems," www.eegspectrum.com/onepage/adhd. htm;

Dr. Seigfried Othmer & Susan Othmer (October, 1992). EEG Biofeedback for Attention Deficit Hyperactivity Disorder; www.eegspectrum.com.

Dr. Bryan Post (2002). Family-Centered Regulatory Therapy. Article published on his website at www.bryanpost.com/fcrt/htm.

Dr. Bryan Post (2002). Video series: Raising Trauma: Understanding, Parenting, and Treating Foster and Adopted Children. www.bryan-post.com.

Beth Powell, LMSW-ACP (1999). Presentation entitled, "Video games and TV shows: What's rot...what's not." Child-in-Family Services: Conroe, TX.

Dan Powers, Doctor of Chiropractic (February 13, 2002). From a seminar entitled, "Complementary Drug-Free Treatments for Symptoms of ADD/ADHD" with The Brain Network.

Stephen C. Putnam (2001). Nature's Ritalin for the Marathon Mind: Nurturing Your ADHD Child with Exercise. Upper Access Book Publishers: Hinesburg, VT.

Judyth Reichenberg-Ullman, N.D., M.S.W., & Robert Ullman, N.D. (1996). Ritalin Free Kids: Safe and Effective Homeopathic Medicine for ADD and Other Behavioral and Learning Problems. Prima Health/ Prima Publishing, CA.

Judyth Reichenberg-Ullman, N.D., L.C.S.W., D.H.A.N.P. & Robert Ullman, N.D., D.H.A.N.P. (2000). Ritalin Free Kids: Safe and Effective Homeopathic Medicine for ADHD and Other Behavioral and Learning Problems, Revised 2nd Edition. Three Rivers Press, NY. Northwest Center for Homeopathic Medicine, 131 3rd Avenue, N., Edmonds, WA, 98020. Tel: (425) 774-5599. www.ritalinfreekids.com

Lauren Robins (2003). The Palette of Breath: Facts About Breathing. Body Sense Press: Wimberley, TX.

Thomas Rossiter & Theodore LaVaque (1995). A comparison of EEG biofeedback and psychostimulants in treating Attention Deficit/ Hyperactivity Disorders, Journal of Neurotherapy, vol. 7(1).

S. Schoenthaler, J. Moody, & L. Pankow (1991). Applied nutrition and behavior. Journal of Applied Nutrition, vol. 43.

Robert Sinaiko, M.D. (1996). Medical Management of Attentional and Behavioral Difficulties of Childhood: Stimulant and Non-Stimulant Strategies, A brief literature review. www.diet-studies.com/review_sinaiko.html.

Ed Smith (1999). Therapeutic Herb Manual: A Guide to the Safe and Effective Use of Liquid Herbal Extracts. Ed Smith, Publisher: Williams, Oregon.

David B. Stein, Ph.D. (1999). Ritalin Is Not The Answer: A Drug-Free, Practical Program for Children Diagnosed with ADD or ADHD. Jossey-Bass Inc., Publishers, CA.

Laura Stevens (2000), 12 Effective Ways to Help Your ADD/ADHD Child, Avery: NY.

Susan Stockton (1990). ADD: It Doesn't Add Up! Nature's Publishing & Printing, Ltd.: FL.

Texas Institute for Rehabilitation and Research, and the Houston Health and Human Services, "Television and Violence."

The ADD/AD/HD Newsletter.
www.attentiondeficitdisorder.ws.

The Brown University Child and Adolescent Psychopharmacology Update (2001). "Monitoring Effects of Drugs: NIMH-led initiative looks to standardize adverse event reporting," volume 3(12).

The Green Guide (2001). Shoppers Guide to Plastics and Food, vol. 8. Published by Mothers and Others for a Livable Planet. www.mothers.org.

T. Uhlig, A. Merkenschlager, R. Brandmaier, & J. Egger (1997). Topographic mapping of brain electrical activity in children with food-induced attention deficit hyperkinetic disorder. European Journal of Pediatrics, vol. 156(7).

Dr. Titus Venessa, Ph.D., Sc.D. (Summer, 2001). "Ask The Expert: ADD." Whole Health System: Lifeline; Newsletter published by Tree of Life: St. Augustine, FL.

Arturo Volpe, D.O. (2001). "Natural Treatments for ADD and AD/HD," seminar, Houston, TX.

Dr. J.D. Wallach, DVM, ND, & Dr. Ma Lan, MD, MS (1998). Let's Play Doctor. Wellness Publications.

Larry Webster (1988). The Hyperactive Child and Chiropractic, Today's Chiropractic, vol. 17(1).

Dr. Walter C. Willett (2001). Eat, Drink, and Be Healthy. Simon & Schuster: New York, NY.

Dr. Tom Williams, Ph.D. (1996). The Complete Illustrated Guide to Chinese Medicine: A Comprehensive System for Health and Fitness. Barnes & Noble Books: New York, NY.

Fan Ya-li (1999). Chinese Pediatric Massage Therapy. Blue Poppy Press: Boulder, CO.

D. Gary Young, N.D. (2001). An Introduction to Young Living Essential Oils (Ninth Edition). Young Living Essential Oils: Payson, UT.

JM Zito, et al. (2000). Trends in prescribing psychotropic medications to preschoolers. Journal of the American Medical Association, vol. 283.

INDEXARY

Acupuncture (See also Chinese Acupuncture): a form of therapy in which special hair-thin needles are used to stimulate specific points on the body as a way of relieving tension and unblocking energy: p. 171, **173-175**

Acupressure (See also Tuí Na): an alternative to Chinese acupuncture; a form of therapy in which the thumbs or fingers are used to apply pressure to specific points on the body as a way of relieving tension and unblocking energy: p. 172, **174**-175

AD/HD (See Attention-Deficit/Hyperactivity Disorder): a diagnosis in the Diagnostic and Statistical Manual of Mental Disorders created and maintained by the American Psychiatric Association, in which children's behavior is described as some combination of impulsive, inattentive, and hyperactive: p. 9

Allopathic Doctor: a licensed physician trained in the medical sciences and emergency procedures, who practices a modern Western (or allopathic) approach to health: p. 23, 188, 196, 210, 235

Allopathic Medicine: the modern Western approach to health that involves the doctor as expert, with a general focus on prescription drugs and/or surgery to treat symptoms, and little emphasis on prevention (although this varies with the individual practitioner): p. 23, 28, 188

Alternative Responses: a form of self-management that involves doing something in place of a behavior that you want to decrease: p. 80

Anderson, Nina: p. 103, 265, 267, 277

Armstrong, Dr. Thomas: p. 146, 159, 160, 266, 267, 277

Aromatherapy: the use of essential plant oils to encourage the body to tap into its self-healing powers: p. 216
Choosing essential plant oils: p. 224
Effectiveness: p. 222
For symptoms of AD/HD: p. 223
Historical uses: p. 217
How it works: p. 218
Modern day uses: p. 217
Safety: p. 221
Using the oils: p. 226

Attention-Deficit/Hyperactivity Disorder (AD/HD): p. 9
Common and uncommon AD/HD drug side effects: p. 19
Criteria for diagnosing AD/HD: p. 10-11
Does AD/HD exist as a unique "disorder?": p. 16
How: Concerns about drug treatments: p. 18
What: AD/HD from the beginning: p. 9
Why revisit the AD/HD diagnosis: p.3
Why: Questions about the cause of AD/HD: p. 14

Axline, Dr. Virginia M. (See also Play Therapy): p. 91, 267, 277

Behavioral Shaping: a tool used to support children in learning a new behaviors: p. 69

Biofeedback: a system of using feedback from sensors attached to different parts of the body to shift your brain waves and/or your body's physiological responses to patterns that will benefit you the most in a given situation: p. **155**, 197, 240, 264, 270, 271
Choosing a biofeedback specialist: p. 161
Effectiveness: p. 157
Safety: p. 157

ENDNOTES

1   Dr. Mary Ann Block (1996). *No More Ritalin: Treating ADHD Without Drugs*, pg. 41. Kensington Books, Kensington Publishing Corp.: NY.

2   Dr. Bryan Post (2002). Video series: Raising Trauma: Understanding, Parenting, and Treating Foster and Adopted Children. www.bryanpost.com.

3   Virginia M. Axline (1947). *Play Therapy*, p. 9. Ballantine Books, Publishers: NY.

4   Nina Anderson & Howard Peiper (1996). *A.D.D.: The Natural Approach*, p. 18. Safe Goods: East Canaan, CT.

5   Dr. Tom Williams, Ph.D. (1996). *The Complete Illustrated Guide to Chinese Medicine: A Comprehensive System for Health and Fitness*, p. 131, 189. Barnes & Noble Books: NY.

6   Michael Sacks, M.D. (1993). In Daniel Goleman, Ph.D., & Joel Gurin (Editors), *Mind Body Medicine: How to Use Your Mind for Better Health*, p. 325. Consumer Reports Books: Yonkers, NY.

7   Judyth Reichenberg-Ullman, N.D., M.S.W., & Robert Ullman, N.D. (1996). Ritalin Free Kids: Safe and Effective Homeopathic Medicine for ADD and Other Behavioral and Learning Problems, p. 26-27. Prima Health, Prima Publishing, CA.

8   Dr. Thomas Armstrong (1995). *The Myth of the A.D.D Child*, p. 76. Plume, NY.

9   Judyth Reichenberg-Ullman, N.D., M.S.W., & Robert Ullman, N.D. (1996). Ritalin Free Kids: Safe and Effective Homeopathic Medicine for ADD and Other Behavioral and Learning Problems, p. 62. Prima Health, Prima Publishing, CA.

10   Judyth Reichenberg-Ullman, N.D., M.S.W., & Robert Ullman, N.D. (1996). Ritalin Free Kids: Safe and Effective Homeopathic Medicine for ADD and Other Behavioral and Learning Problems, p. 80. Prima Health, Prima Publishing, CA.

[11] Dr. James Duke (1997). *The Green Pharmacy*, p.2. Rodale Press: Emmaus, PA.

[12] Carolyn L. Mein, D.C. (1998). *Releasing Emotional Patterns with Essential Oils*, p. 5. Rancho Santa Fe, CA.